T0205482

The Unified Airway

David A. Gudis • Rodney J. Schlosser

Editors

The Unified Airway

Rhinologic Disease and Respiratory Disorders

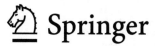 Springer

Editors
David A. Gudis
Otolaryngology – Head & Neck Surgery
Columbia University
New York, NY
USA

Rodney J. Schlosser
Otolaryngology - Head and Neck Surgery
Medical University of South Carolina
Charleston, SC
USA

ISBN 978-3-030-50332-1   ISBN 978-3-030-50330-7   (eBook)
https://doi.org/10.1007/978-3-030-50330-7

This Springer imprint is published by the registered company Springer Nature Switzerland AG
The registered company address is: Gewerbestrasse 11, 6330 Cham, Switzerland

To my patients, whose courage, strength, and trust truly inspires and humbles me.
To Rod, a phenomenal mentor and friend.
To my wife Charlotte and my daughters Isabelle and Eloise, whose love and support allows me to love going to work and love coming home.

–David A. Gudis, MD

To my wife Chris for her unconditional love.
To my sons Nate and Steve for the joy they bring to my life.
To colleagues, staff, and patients who let me play a part in their lives.
To God for all these blessings and many more.

–Rodney J. Schlosser, MD

Foreword

The concept of the unified airway, the interplay between the upper and lower airway, has been around for over 20 years, and it is very gratifying to have a book which takes a holistic approach to this well-recognized relationship. This new book expands this original concept to discuss the connection between chronic rhinosinusitis (CRS) and many other important comorbid respiratory diseases. The original unified airway studies demonstrated that when the upper airway was challenged with allergen, an inflammatory response also occurred in the lower airway and vice versa, proving that the inflammatory response in one part of the unified airways could cause an inflammation in another part of the same airway. Epidemiological studies have confirmed this connection, and it has been shown that 80% or more of asthma patients have allergic rhinitis (AR) and 40% of AR patients have asthma. Similarly, the relationship between CRS and lower airway disease such as bronchiectasis and COPD has increasingly become a focus of attention. Further, recent studies have demonstrated that surgical and medical management of CRS not only improves asthma but can also delay and perhaps even avoid the onset of asthma. These concepts emphasize the importance of this relationship between upper and lower airways.

This book, edited by some of the leaders in the field, and with book chapters each of which is written by an expert in that particular aspect of the problem, coalesces each of the disorders and the relationships identified between the upper and lower airways, particularly in relationship to CRS. Within this context, the book explores such issues as bronchiectasis and chronic rhinosinusitis, cystic fibrosis, aspirin exacerbated respiratory disease (AERD), asthma, and allergic rhinitis, making this important reading for practicing otolaryngologists, allergists, and residents alike. This text highlights the importance of seeing the patient as a whole, rather than looking at airway diseases as separate entities treated by different specialists. The result is to emphasize the need to collaborate very closely with our pulmonology and allergy colleagues so as to understand how these diseases interact and effect patients' health as a whole. This book does a great work of highlighting these interactions. For instance, the chapter on bronchiectasis points out that, in one study, patients with bronchiectasis had a 62% prevalence of co-morbid CRS.

The *one airway* concept is central to our understanding of the need to manage even minimally symptomatic or asymptomatic upper airway disease. Thus, it is critical that all otolaryngologists and allergists are fully aware of these relationships uniting the upper and lower airway in an inseparable bond. This book therefore makes essential reading for those involved in each of these fields.

David W Kennedy, MD, FRCSI, FACS
Elina M Toskala, MD, MBA, PhD

Preface

Since Hippocrates first described asthma in the fifth century BC, physicians and surgeons have struggled to understand the deep complexities of inflammatory airway disorders. The earliest descriptions of removing nasal polyps in patients with asthma, over a century ago, represent early explorations into the mysteries of the unified airway. However, it has taken thousands of years for doctors and scientists to uncover the intricate relationship between the upper and lower airway.

Fortunately, in the last few decades, tremendous strides have been taken along this road of discovery. Among clinicians, there is now a true appreciation for the unified airway, and it is now recognized that most – if not all – inflammatory disorders that impact one airway subsite have similar effects throughout the entire airway. Similarly, we now understand that medical and surgical interventions for one airway subsite can likewise benefit the entire airway and, indeed, a patient's systemic health.

Appreciation of the unified airway has led to dramatic improvements for our patients. The approach to patients with chronic rhinosinusitis now includes considerations regarding lower airway disease. These patients are often treated by multidisciplinary teams, and clinical trials typically investigate both upper and lower airway effects of a given therapeutic intervention. It is an exciting time to care for these patients when one is armed with the knowledge that sinus surgery may reduce the required maintenance therapy for an asthma patient or reduce lung infections for a cystic fibrosis patient.

We hope that this text will further advance the understanding of the important link between rhinologic disease and respiratory disorders in the unified airway.

New York, NY, USA David A. Gudis
Charleston, SC, USA Rodney J. Schlosser

Contents

Contributors

Kasper Aanaes Department of Otorhinolaryngology Head and Neck Surgery and Audiology, Copenhagen University Hospital, Rigshospitalet, Copenhagen, Denmark

Waleed M. Abuzeid Division of Rhinology and Skull Base Surgery, Department of Otolaryngology: Head and Neck Surgery, University of Washington, Seattle, WA, USA

Mikkel Christian Alanin Department of Otorhinolaryngology, Rigshospitalet, Copenhagen, Denmark

Catherine Banks Department of Otolaryngology-Head and Neck Surgery, Prince of Wales and Sydney Hospitals, University of New South Wales, Randwick, Sydney, NSW, Australia

Ryan Belcher Surgical Outcomes Center for Kids (SOCKs), Vanderbilt University Medical Center, Nashville, TN, USA

Department of Otolaryngology-Head & Neck Surgery, Vanderbilt University Medical Center, Nashville, TN, USA

Monroe Carell Jr. Children's Hospital at Vanderbilt, Nashville, TN, USA

John V. Bosso Division of Rhinology, Department of Otorhinolaryngology, Head and Neck Surgery, Perelman School of Medicine, University of Pennsylvania, Philadelphia, PA, USA

Do-Yeon Cho Department of Otolaryngology Head and Neck Surgery, University of Alabama at Birmingham School of Medicine, Birmingham, AL, USA

Gregory Fleming James Cystic Fibrosis Research Center, Birmingham, AL, USA

John M. DelGaudio Department of Otolaryngology – Head and Neck Surgery, Emory University, Atlanta, GA, USA

Thomas S. Edwards Department of Otolaryngology – Head and Neck Surgery, Emory University, Atlanta, GA, USA

Jarret Foster University of South Carolina School of Medicine, Columbia, SC, USA

Surgical Outcomes Center for Kids (SOCKs), Vanderbilt University Medical Center, Nashville, TN, USA

Sarah A. Gitomer Otolaryngology – Head and Neck Surgery, Children's Hospital Colorado, Aurora, CO, USA

Jessica W. Grayson Department of Otolaryngology Head and Neck Surgery, University of Alabama at Birmingham School of Medicine, Birmingham, AL, USA

David A. Gudis Department of Otolaryngology – Head & Neck Surgery, Columbia University Irving Medical Center, NewYork-Presbyterian Hospital, New York, NY, USA

Sukaina Hasnie Department of Otolaryngology – Head and Neck Surgery, University of Oklahoma College of Medicine, Oklahoma City, OK, USA

Samuel N. Helman Department of Otolaryngology – Head and Neck Surgery, Emory University, Atlanta, GA, USA

Kevin Hur Department of Otolaryngology - Head and Neck Surgery, Feinberg School of Medicine, Northwestern University, Chicago, IL, USA

Peter H. Hwang Division of Endoscopic Sinus & Skull Base Surgery, Department of Otolaryngology-Head & Neck Surgery, Stanford University School of Medicine, Stanford, CA, USA

Raymond Kim Division of Endoscopic Sinus & Skull Base Surgery, Department of Otolaryngology-Head & Neck Surgery, Stanford University School of Medicine, Stanford, CA, USA

Kevin Li Department of Otorhinolaryngology: Head and Neck Surgery, Division of Rhinology and Skull Base Surgery, Montefiore Medical Center, Albert Einstein College of Medicine, Bronx, NY, USA

Brittany Lipscomb Surgical Outcomes Center for Kids (SOCKs), Vanderbilt University Medical Center, Nashville, TN, USA

Department of Otolaryngology-Head & Neck Surgery, Vanderbilt University Medical Center, Nashville, TN, USA

Daljit S. Mann Department of Otolaryngology – Head and Neck Surgery, University of Oklahoma College of Medicine, Oklahoma City, OK, USA

Kibwei A. McKinney Department of Otolaryngology – Head and Neck Surgery, University of Oklahoma College of Medicine, Oklahoma City, OK, USA

Jonathan Overdevest Department of Otolaryngology – Head & Neck Surgery, Columbia University Irving Medical Center, NewYork-Presbyterian Hospital, New York, NY, USA

Viraj Patel Department of Otorhinolaryngology: Head and Neck Surgery, Division of Rhinology and Skull Base Surgery, Montefiore Medical Center, Albert Einstein College of Medicine, Bronx, NY, USA

Vijay Ramakrishnan Department of Otolaryngology, University of Colorado School of Medicine, Aurora, CO, USA

Chetan Safi Department of Otolaryngology – Head & Neck Surgery, Columbia University Irving Medical Center, NewYork-Presbyterian Hospital, New York, NY, USA

Daniel Spielman Department of Otolaryngology – Head & Neck Surgery, Columbia University Irving Medical Center, NewYork-Presbyterian Hospital, New York, NY, USA

Auddie M. Sweis Division of Rhinology, Department of Otorhinolaryngology, Head and Neck Surgery, Perelman School of Medicine, University of Pennsylvania, Philadelphia, PA, USA

Harrison Thompson Department of Otolaryngology Head and Neck Surgery, University of Alabama at Birmingham School of Medicine, Birmingham, AL, USA

Frank W. Virgin Surgical Outcomes Center for Kids (SOCKs), Vanderbilt University Medical Center, Nashville, TN, USA

Department of Otolaryngology-Head & Neck Surgery, Vanderbilt University Medical Center, Nashville, TN, USA

Monroe Carell Jr. Children's Hospital at Vanderbilt, Nashville, TN, USA

Kevin C. Welch Department of Otolaryngology – Head and Neck Surgery, Feinberg School of Medicine, Northwestern University, Chicago, IL, USA

Sarah K. Wise Department of Otolaryngology – Head and Neck Surgery, Emory University, Atlanta, GA, USA

Bradford A. Woodworth Gregory Fleming James Cystic Fibrosis Research Center, Birmingham, AL, USA

Department of Otolaryngology-Head and Neck Surgery, University of Alabama at Birmingham, Birmingham, AL, USA

Chapter 1
Microbiome of the Unified Airway

Sarah A. Gitomer and Vijay Ramakrishnan

> **Key Concepts**
> - The human microbiome influences airway physiology, including both downregulation and activation of inflammatory cascades.
> - Patients with CRS have distinct features of their microbial community architecture.
> - The therapeutic role of probiotics remains an area of active investigation.

It has long been recognized that numerous diverse microbes colonize the human body and that microbial cells greatly outnumber eukaryotic cells [1]. In the past 20 years, the variety of microbial communities and their genes became defined as the microbiome, and research into the interactions between hosts and resident microbiomes has exploded [2]. Variations in the microbiome have been implicated in a variety of disease processes, from autism, to cardiovascular disease, to cancer [3, 4]. Its role in mucosal inflammation in organ systems connected to the outer world is most strongly implicated, and research into the sinonasal, laryngeal, and pulmonary microbiota in health and disease is growing. Considering the physical connection, similar exposures, cell types, and immune response in airway sites, it is not surprising that bacterial communities are similar throughout the entire airway [5]. In fact, these similarities create the foundation for the unified airway hypothesis.

S. A. Gitomer
Otolaryngology—Head and Neck Surgery, Children's Hospital Colorado, Aurora, CO, USA
e-mail: sarah.gitomer@childrenscolorado.org

V. Ramakrishnan (✉)
Department of Otolaryngology, University of Colorado School of Medicine,
Aurora, CO, USA
e-mail: vijay.ramakrishnan@cuanschutz.edu

© Springer Nature Switzerland AG 2020
D. A. Gudis, R. J. Schlosser (eds.), *The Unified Airway*,
https://doi.org/10.1007/978-3-030-50330-7_1

1

Research Techniques

Our knowledge and understanding of the microbiome have evolved alongside technological innovations. First, investigations into the bacterial communities lining the gastrointestinal tract relied on culture-based identification of the microbes in various locations [1]. However, traditional cultures are limited because they rely on the ability to reproduce specific niche characteristics of the human body in a laboratory [6]. Therefore, scientists turned to "culture-independent" techniques that proved more sensitive than traditional culture, and these techniques permitted identification of organisms that otherwise would not be identified with *in vitro* cultures [6, 7]. As polymerase chain reaction (PCR) technology evolved, researchers turned to restriction fragment length polymorphism (RFLP), a DNA-based technology that compares specific sequences of DNA in a sample to known profiles for specific bacteria [8]. In order to better understand bacterial communities, researchers capitalized on the unique 16S subunit of bacterial ribosomal rRNA. By amplifying and sequencing segments of this rRNA, scientists are able to identify the unique genetic fingerprint of each bacterium and quantify how much is present in a sample [6, 7]. The newest evolution of this technology sequences the full-length 16S rRNA genes in order to obtain species-level details about resident bacteria [9]. Whole-genome shotgun sequencing provides more data about individual microbes, providing enhanced detection of bacterial species and the possibility of understanding how genetic differences within each species of bacteria may drive changes in the microbiome-host interaction in health and disease [10]. With the amount of data generated with each technique and the vast differences seen between individuals even in healthy states, making microbiome comparisons across patients must be done with great care.

This area of research is further complicated by the fact that different niches within the body harbor unique collections of microbes [3, 11–13] and that different sampling techniques may lead to different results. This research has been criticized by concerns that sampling techniques bias the results and that contamination by the nasal or oral cavity influences results from deeper subsites [14, 15]. However, several studies have shown that there is continuity of the microbial profiles throughout the airway [14–16]. In health, microbial populations in the oral cavity, oropharynx, larynx, and lungs are very similar within each individual [14]. In chronic rhinosinusitis (CRS), sampling each sinus independently shows that each sinus may have some differences in bacterial composition, but that anatomic subsites within the sinonasal cavity do not represent a major source of differences in microbiota [16]. Furthermore, the anterior nares and the paranasal sinuses have been shown to have very similar microbiota, both in healthy controls and in CRS patients [15]. However, inter-patient variation is significant, and individuals suffering from the same disease have significantly different microbial fingerprints [16, 17]. The varying physiology of different anatomic subsites likely accounts for the biggest changes seen in the microbiome, sometimes more so than separation by distance [18, 19].

Future Directions

The current focus in this field has been on the role of bacteria, but there is novel research investigating the overall pathobiome: how viruses, fungi, archaea, and other pathogens influence health and disease [20–23]. In order to better understand host responses to alterations in the microbiome, metagenomic approaches are also being used to characterize how functional networks drive chronic airway diseases [24].

Overall, microbiome research is a relatively young field with several exciting opportunities for discovery. However, as we sort through the enormous amount of data produced and understand the limitations of techniques, the clinical practice implications remain in their infancy. Current research is promising but is still far from direct patient impact [25]. This chapter summarizes the current understanding of the microbiome in the unified airway. Because each individual and disease process are so unique, we focus on distinct representative patterns in this chapter: microbiome variations in allergic airway disease (CRS and asthma), cystic fibrosis, and the gut-airway axis.

Etiology and Pathogenesis

Bacteria present throughout the airway help regulate health, prevent disease, or may alternatively lead to chronic inflammation and disease states. Microbes influence the host by modulating the immune system, changing the epithelial barrier, and competing or cooperating with other microbiomes to maintain or disrupt healthy equilibrium. Commensal bacteria in the oral cavity suppress inflammation by modulating Toll-like receptor signaling or NF-Kß inhibition, while others prime the immune system to improve inflammatory responses to pathogens [26]. Conversely, certain pathogenic bacteria create a pro-inflammatory state in the airway by inducing the production of cytokines, and the impacts of this imbalance can be synergistic. For instance, when *Streptococcus pneumoniae* and *Haemophilus influenzae* co-colonize airway epithelium *in vivo* and *in vitro*, they activate a significant inflammatory pathway that is more pronounced than when either is present in isolation [27]. Microbes throughout the airway can influence the epithelial barrier integrity which may be a key driver of inflammation seen in asthma [28]. Furthermore, bacteria within each niche compete with and modulate the growth of other bacteria [25]. For example, *Staphylococcus lugdunensis*, *S. epidermidis*, and *Corynebacterium pseudodiphtheriticum* have been shown *in vitro* to inhibit growth of a known pathogen *S. aureus*, while *C. accolens* has been shown to enhance its growth [29–32]. Therefore, either health or disease is a culmination of numerous and continuous interactions between colonizing bacteria and between bacteria and the immune system—not just a result of a "healthy" or "unhealthy" microbiome.

The Microbiome Shifts over Time

The initial colonization of the airway microbiome begins at birth, and changes have been identified based on vaginal versus caesarian delivery. Upper airway colonization undergoes the most change during the first year of life [33]. At birth, the nasopharyngeal microbiome most resembles either the vaginal or skin microbiome depending on the delivery method. In otherwise healthy breastfed infants, this flora stays relatively constant, with a higher proportion of bacteria that are theorized to be protective against respiratory infections (*Dolosigranulum* and *Corynebacterium*); however, in formula-fed infants, these patterns shift toward increases in *S. aureus* [34, 35]. Over time, the microbiome patterns continue to evolve. Healthy airways display more diverse but less dense bacterial colonization, with unique niches that develop in the various airway subsites [19, 36]. In the elderly, there is a loss of niche specificity, which can predispose older people to opportunistic infections like pneumonia [36, 37].

Living Conditions Influence the Bacterial Colonization of the Airway

In addition to age and early life exposures, there have been several other influences that shape the microbiome. In comparing the anterior nares in healthy German volunteers to the anterior nares of healthy Babongo Pygmy tribe member volunteers, there was an 85% overlap in phylotypes detected between these geographically and culturally distinct populations [38]. This suggests not only that our environment can influence our microbiome but also that the global bacterial communities present in the anterior nares have likely been present for thousands of years—the time when the German and Pygmy tribe volunteers' ancestors lived together [38]. Humans' environment and living conditions also influence the airway microbiome. When examining astronauts living together in the International Space Station for long durations, researchers noted changes within the nasal, skin, and GI bacterial populations within one week of space travel, and these changes persisted for months after returning home [39].

The "Healthy Microbiome"

Overall, complex interactions between host defenses and the microbiome can determine the health of the host. The basic principle of microbiome theory is that when both host and microbes are living in a commensal state, patients remain healthy, but when this state is disrupted (i.e., dysbiosis), commensal bacteria are replaced by opportunistic pathogens which can lead to diseases such as inflammatory bowel disease, obesity, diabetes, and chronic rhinosinusitis [40–44]. Based on this concept, scientists have searched for the "healthy" microbiome—a collection of commensal bacteria that help maintain healthy homeostasis. However, each individual has a different microbial fingerprint during health and illness, making one specific set of protective airway bacteria difficult to define [45]. However, some patterns have emerged. The most commonly identified bacteria in the healthy sinonasal microbiome are members from the genera *Propionibacterium*, Actinobacteria, Bacteroidetes, Firmicutes, Proteobacteria with representatives of genera *Bifidobacterium*, *Corynebacterium*, *Staphylococcus*, *Streptococcus*, *Dolosigranulum*, and *Moraxella* predominating [19, 36, 46, 47]. It should be noted that certain bacteria that are generally considered pathogens (such as *S. aureus*) are commonly identified in healthy patients, suggesting that changes within the bacteria themselves (increased abundance, acquisition and expression of virulence genes, etc.) or the host response may be more important than the species' presence or absence in in the airway. The relationship between human airway disease and the associated dysbiosis is challenging to define because it is not known if microbiota changes represent the underlying disease etiology, are simply a sign of disease, or are a by-product of disease therapies [25].

Clinical Presentation

Because microbiome study is so broad and complex and there are significant effects in almost every disease process in the unified airway, this chapter focuses on commonly identified themes. Because many airway diseases have similar inflammatory pathways and similar treatments including steroids and antibiotics, similar changes in the microbiome may be observed throughout the airway.

Atopic Airway Diseases: Allergic Rhinitis, Chronic Rhinosinusitis, and Asthma

Allergic rhinitis (AR), chronic rhinosinusitis (CRS), and asthma are atopic diseases that are commonly associated [48]. CRS is a heterogeneous clinical syndrome characterized by significant sinonasal inflammation leading to similar symptoms. The underlying etiology is thought to be multifactorial, but the exact underlying mechanism remains unclear [45]. Several factors including allergens, host immunodeficiency, and microbes have been investigated [45, 49, 50]. Asthma is similarly a chronic disease characterized by airway inflammation and hyperresponsiveness where long-term recurrent episodes of inflammation can lead to airway remodeling [51]. To be sure, some CRS and asthma subtypes may not be atopic in nature. While these diseases have similar presentations and triggers, the changes observed in the microbiome are different.

While CRS may consist of numerous subtypes with distinct clinical courses and exam findings, consistent patterns have been observed. Although the overall bacterial burden is similar in health and disease, patients with CRS have less biodiversity detected in sinus samples than healthy controls or in patients with AR [45, 52, 53]. CRS patients generally have more abundant anaerobes, *S. aureus*, and members of the genus *Corynebacterium* detected than healthy controls do [40, 54]. CRS patients have also been found to cluster into distinct subgroups with different host responses that correlate with disease severity [55]. Despite the unified airway, patients with CRS maintain unique microbial communities compared to lung samples, implying that in this disease process, the sinuses and lungs maintain distinct microbial niches [56].

Conversely, more diversity in the microbiome is associated with worse asthma [57–59]. In particular, asthmatics have more Proteobacteria including Comamonadaceae, Sphingomonadaceae, Nitrosomonadaceae, Oxalobacteraceae, and Pseudomonadaceae families. However, similar to the sinuses, the presence of *Actinobacteria* is associated with improved asthma control [58].

Cystic Fibrosis

Unique alterations to the airway microbiome are detected early in CF [60]. Neonates with CF have distinct nasal and nasopharyngeal bacterial loads compared to healthy controls, in particular Staphylococcaceae even before exposure to any antibiotics [61, 62]. Even before age 8, bronchial alveolar lavage (BAL) specimens from CF patients are distinct from healthy controls in that CF patients host *Corynebacterium* and *Streptococcus* species in this young age group [63]. Older children and adults with CF are consistently found to have less diversity of the lung microbiome compared to healthy controls, with certain pathogenic bacteria predominating the community [63, 64]. Over time, the pulmonary bacteria become even less diverse, and adults with CF are found to have overgrowth of a single pathogen compared to the diverse colonization seen in younger CF children [65]. Although individual CF patients may have taxonomic differences in the predominant microbes detected in the airways, studies have shown that these different populations have similar functional consequences [66]. This is clinically relevant because decreased microbiome diversity is associated with worse pulmonary function and worse disease compared to controls [67–70].

Unlike allergic airways, the unified airway in CF is found to have similar populations in the upper and lower airways. The microbial fingerprint of the saliva and oropharynx is found to be more similar to the sputum cultures from the same child with CF than similar subsites in other children but underrepresents the bacterial load [62, 71]. Similarly, adults with CF have similar bacterial populations detected in the sinuses and the lungs [56]. The loss of niche specificity in the CF airway is notable and may reflect the underlying innate immune dysfunction in this disease. As the upper and lower airways' bacterial populations diverge, there is more evidence of lung damage and more severe disease, suggesting expansion of pathogenic bacteria in the lungs unaccompanied by changes in the oropharynx is correlated with pulmonary injury [71].

Gut-Airway Axis

There has been some investigation into the role of changes in the gastrointestinal (GI) microbiome in influencing inflammatory patterns seen in the airway [72]. It is hypothesized that early colonization of the gut microbiome primes the immune system, and variations in the intestinal microbes have been linked with several inflammatory diseases, including autoimmune disease [73, 74]. Similarly, it is hypothesized that the gut microbiota may influence airway diseases. Early alterations in GI bacteria (such as increases in *Clostridium difficile* or *E. coli*) have been seen to precede diagnosis with atopy or eczema later in childhood, while patients with more stable early communities do not go on to develop atopy (including AR) [75, 76]. In mouse models, early colonization of the gut with *Lactobacillus johnsonii* is correlated with protection from asthma [77]. As seen in their airway, adult patients with CF have decreased bacterial diversity in the GI tract compared to healthy controls [78]. When investigated in a serial manner in infants with CF, alterations in the gut microbiome preceded and predicted similar changes and development of specific bacteria in the airways. Furthermore, as the infants' diets progressed, changes are seen in the GI and then airway microbiomes [79]. This etiologic connection has not been thoroughly studied in CRS, although the relationship between GI and airway microbiomes represents another pathway for understanding the heterogeneous inflammation seen in this disease.

Molecular Diagnostic Tools in Clinical Practice

Recent translational research has described the use of culture-independent techniques in clinical practice. Some authors have described next-generation sequencing (NGS) as a complement to traditional microbiology laboratory studies but, given the limited understanding of the sinonasal microbiome, advised against its routine use in clinical practice at this time [80]. Retrospective reviews have reported the use of this technology to characterize acute exacerbations of CRS with more comprehensive identification and quantification of bacteria present, yet the clinical utility of these tests is unclear, in part due to the lack of functional evaluation of antimicrobial susceptibilities [81]. Compared to standard diagnosis with computed tomography scans, DNA sequencing has a high negative predictive value (99.1%) but low positive predictive value (19.4%) of an odontogenic source of CRS [82]. In clinical practice, culture-independent diagnostics identify the same bacteria detected with traditional culture in addition to other predominant organisms that are not found with cultures. Clinical outcomes and utility are yet to be defined, but culture-independent microbiota diagnostics have been suggested as a potential tool for patients with recalcitrant CRS in order to improve antimicrobial treatment [83].

Medical Management and Outcomes: Alternatives to Antibiotics

As research efforts continue to define the relationship between airway disease and the microbiome, there is much hope that this information will lead to novel therapeutics that target airway inflammation while reducing reliance on antibiotics. In GI disease, such interventions have already demonstrated benefit: oral probiotics can reduce complications and disease severity in hospitalized adults receiving antibiotics for *C. difficile* [84]. The systemic and local administration of therapeutic probiotics for airway disease has been investigated, with varying levels of evidence supporting efficacy at this time.

Systemic Medical Therapy

Most evidence for the use of oral probiotics in airway disease comes from studies examining their use in preventing respiratory viral infections, harnessing the gut-airway axis. Well-designed trials have shown that oral probiotics decrease the frequency and severity of upper respiratory tract infections (URIs) and acute sinusitis in children and the elderly [85–87]. A systematic review confirmed that in immunocompetent children, there is modest decrease in severity and/or incidence of URIs with prophylactic probiotic administration [88]. Probiotic milk during pregnancy and early childhood has been associated with decreased rate of rhinoconjunctivitis and eczema, but no difference was seen in the rate of asthma by age 3 years [89]. Similarly, in pilot data, prophylactic oral probiotics for CF patients have been correlated with decreased number of pulmonary exacerbations [90]. Overall, there is growing support for the use of oral systemic probiotics to prevent acute infections, but their use in chronic airway disease is not yet well-studied [91].

Topical Medical Therapy

Topical probiotics have been investigated in the use of mitigating unified airway diseases. Preclinical data modeling the topical use of gram-positive bacteria shows that such treatments may be safe for epithelial cells and induce anti-inflammatory cytokine responses [92]. One described technique is to use specific bacteria to target underlying sources of inflammation in chronic airway disease. For instance, *S. salivarius* and *S. oralis* disrupt upper airway biofilms and could represent a tailored topical probiotic for the treatment of CRS [93]. In animal models of allergic asthma, intranasal *L. rhamnosus* use is correlated to decreased BAL inflammatory markers that initiate asthma attacks, suggesting a targeted approach for decreasing pulmonary hyperreactivity [94]. Because our knowledge of the dysbiosis seen in CRS remains in its infancy, with limited information about causation, some investigators have argued that much larger and more thorough clinical trials are warranted prior to standard use of topical probiotics in CRS [95].

Impact of Rhinologic Interventions on the Microbiome

Both medical and surgical therapy for CRS influence the sinonasal microbiome. Topical medications including steroids and antibiotics shift the diversity of bacterial populations, and these effects persist beyond the duration of treatment [96]. Similarly, nasal saline irrigation has been shown to decrease the microbial burden in the sinuses [97]. Immediately after endoscopic sinus surgery and postoperative antibiotic therapy, the overall bacterial burden in the sinuses is relatively unchanged, but the types of bacteria present shift to a varying degree. Then, 6 weeks postoperatively, the microbiome reverts to a population similar to the preoperative colonization in many subjects [98]. The use of perioperative medications, disruption of mucociliary clearance, and traumatic inflammation associated with surgery may all impact these changes. However, it is worth noting that the degree of stability and resilience to major intervention varies among patients. Therefore, intentional microbiome manipulation may not be equally achievable in all people. Even the size of maxillary antrostomy has been associated with differences in the postoperative sinus microbiome, although the relevance of this is unknown [99]. It is critical to recognize that therapeutic interventions are associated with significant changes in the sinonasal microbiome, but the colonization patterns exhibit some degree of resilience, and many confounders limit the understanding of causality.

Conclusion

The microbiome of the unified airway remains an active area of investigation. Though the field is in its infancy, our current understanding of the airway microbiome suggests that the microbiome is a major factor of airway function both in health and in disease. The translational and clinical applications of this emerging scientific discovery remain unclear, but therapeutic interventions to influence the microbiome may have a role in future CRS management.

References

1. Savage DC. Microbial ecology of the gastrointestinal tract. Annu Rev Microbiol [Internet]. 1977 Oct [cited 2020 Jan 26];31(1):107–33. Available from: http://www.annualreviews.org/doi/10.1146/annurev.mi.31.100177.000543.
2. Methé BA, Nelson KE, Pop M, Creasy HH, Giglio MG, Huttenhower C, et al. A framework for human microbiome research. Nature. 2012;486(7402):215–21.

3. Proctor LM, Creasy HH, Fettweis JM, Lloyd-Price J, Mahurkar A, Zhou W, et al. The integrative human microbiome project. Nature. 2019;569(7758):641–8.
4. Integrative HMP Research Network Consortium T. Cell Host & Microbe The Integrative Human Microbiome Project: Dynamic Analysis of Microbiome-Host Omics Profiles during Periods of Human Health and Disease. 2014 [cited 2020 Jan 26]. Available from: https://doi.org/10.1016/j.chom.2014.08.014. ThisisanopenaccessarticleundertheCCBYlicense.
5. Hanshew AS, Jetté ME, Rosen SP, Thibeault SL. Integrating the microbiota of the respiratory tract with the unified airway model, vol. 126: Respiratory Medicine WB Saunders Ltd; 2017. p. 68–74.
6. Ward DM, Weller R, Bateson MM. 16S rRNA sequences reveal numerous uncultured microorganisms in a natural community. Nature. 1990;345(6270):63–5.
7. Vickery TW, Kofonow JM, Ramakrishnan VR. Characterization of sinus microbiota by 16S sequencing from swabs. In: Methods in molecular biology: Humana Press Inc; 2017. p. 23–38.
8. Camarinha-Silva A, Wos-Oxley ML, Jáuregui R, Becker K, Pieper DH. Validating T-RFLP as a sensitive and high-throughput approach to assess bacterial diversity patterns in human anterior nares. FEMS Microbiol Ecol. 2012;79(1):98–108.
9. Earl JP, Adappa ND, Krol J, Bhat AS, Balashov S, Ehrlich RL, et al. Species-level bacterial community profiling of the healthy sinonasal microbiome using Pacific Biosciences sequencing of full-length 16S rRNA genes. Microbiome [Internet]. 2018 [cited 2019 Oct 31];6(1):190. Available from: http://www.ncbi.nlm.nih.gov/pubmed/30352611.
10. Ranjan R, Rani A, Metwally A, McGee HS, Perkins DL. Analysis of the microbiome: advantages of whole genome shotgun versus 16S amplicon sequencing. Biochem Biophys Res Commun [Internet]. 2016 Jan [cited 2020 Jan 26];469(4):967–77. Available from: https://linkinghub.elsevier.com/retrieve/pii/S0006291X15310883.
11. Huttenhower C, Gevers D, Knight R, Abubucker S, Badger JH, Chinwalla AT, et al. Structure, function and diversity of the healthy human microbiome. Nature. 2012;486(7402):207–14.
12. Lloyd-Price J, Mahurkar A, Rahnavard G, Crabtree J, Orvis J, Hall AB, et al. Strains, functions and dynamics in the expanded human microbiome project. Nature. 2017;550(7674):61–6.
13. Peterson J, Garges S, Giovanni M, McInnes P, Wang L, Schloss JA, et al. The NIH human microbiome project. Genome Res. 2009;19(12):2317–23.
14. Charlson ES, Bittinger K, Haas AR, Fitzgerald AS, Frank I, Yadav A, et al. Topographical Continuity of Bacterial Populations in the Healthy Human Respiratory Tract. [cited 2020 Jan 26]. Available from: www.atsjournals.org.
15. De Boeck I, Wittouck S, Martens K, Claes J, Jorissen M, Steelant B, et al. Anterior Nares Diversity and Pathobionts Represent Sinus Microbiome in Chronic Rhinosinusitis. mSphere [Internet]. 2019 Nov 27 [cited 2020 Jan 26];4(6). Available from: http://www.ncbi.nlm.nih.gov/pubmed/31776238.
16. Ramakrishnan VR, Gitomer S, Kofonow JM, Robertson CE, Frank DN. Investigation of sinonasal microbiome spatial organization in chronic rhinosinusitis. Int Forum Allergy Rhinol [Internet]. 2017;7(1):16–23. Available from: http://www.ncbi.nlm.nih.gov/pubmed/27627048.
17. Copeland E, Leonard K, Carney R, Kong J, Forer M, Naidoo Y, et al. Chronic rhinosinusitis: potential role of microbial dysbiosis and recommendations for sampling sites. Front Cell Infect Microbiol. 2018;8(FEB).
18. Proctor DM, Relman DA. The landscape ecology and microbiota of the human nose, mouth, and throat, vol. 21: Cell Host and Microbe. Cell Press; 2017. p. 421–32.
19. Bassis CM, Tang AL, Young VB, Pynnonen MA. The nasal cavity microbiota of healthy adults. Microbiome. 2014;2(1).
20. Koskinen K, Pausan MR, Perras AK, Beck M, Bang C, Mora M, et al. First insights into the diverse human archaeome: specific detection of archaea in the gastrointestinal tract, lung, and nose and on skin. MBio. 2017;8(6).
21. Zhang I, Pletcher SD, Goldberg AN, Barker BM, Cope EK. Fungal microbiota in chronic airway inflammatory disease and emerging relationships with the host immune response. Front Microbiol. 2017;8(DEC).

22. Cleland EJ, Bassioni A, Boase S, Dowd S, Vreugde S, Wormald P-J. The fungal microbiome in chronic rhinosinusitis: richness, diversity, postoperative changes and patient outcomes. Int Forum Allergy Rhinol [Internet]. 2014 Apr;4(4):259–65. Available from: http://doi.wiley.com/10.1002/alr.21297.
23. Goggin RK, Bennett CA, Bassiouni A, Bialasiewicz S, Vreugde S, Wormald PJ, et al. Comparative viral sampling in the sinonasal passages; different viruses at different sites. Front Cell Infect Microbiol. 2018;8(SEP).
24. Altman MC, Gill MA, Whalen E, Babineau DC, Shao B, Liu AH, et al. Transcriptome networks identify mechanisms of viral and nonviral asthma exacerbations in children. Nat Immunol. 2019;20(5):637–51.
25. Kumpitsch C, Koskinen K, Schöpf V, Moissl-Eichinger C. The microbiome of the upper respiratory tract in health and disease. BMC Biol [Internet]. 2019 Dec 7;17(1):87. Available from: https://bmcbiol.biomedcentral.com/articles/10.1186/s12915-019-0703-z.
26. Devine DA, Marsh PD, Meade J. Modulation of host responses by oral commensal bacteria, vol. 7: Journal of Oral Microbiology Co-Action Publishing; 2015. p. 1–4.
27. Ratner AJ, Lysenko ES, Paul MN, Weiser JN. Synergistic proinflammatory responses induced by polymicrobial colonization of epithelial surfaces. Proc Natl Acad Sci U S A. 2005;102(9):3429–34.
28. Georas SN, Rezaee F. Epithelial barrier function: at the front line of asthma immunology and allergic airway inflammation. J Allergy Clin Immunol. 2014;134:509–20.
29. Yan M, Pamp SJ, Fukuyama J, Hwang PH, Cho DY, Holmes S, et al. Nasal microenvironments and interspecific interactions influence nasal microbiota complexity and S. aureus carriage. Cell Host Microbe. 2013;14(6):631–40.
30. Zipperer A, Konnerth MC, Laux C, Berscheid A, Janek D, Weidenmaier C, et al. Human commensals producing a novel antibiotic impair pathogen colonization. Nature. 2016;535(7613):511–6.
31. Ramsey MM, Freire MO, Gabrilska RA, Rumbaugh KP, Lemon KP. Staphylococcus aureus shifts toward commensalism in response to corynebacterium species. Front Microbiol. 2016;7(AUG).
32. Stubbendieck RM, May DS, Chevrette MG, Temkin MI, Wendt-Pienkowski E, Cagnazzo J, et al. Competition among Nasal Bacteria Suggests a Role for Siderophore-Mediated Interactions in Shaping the Human Nasal Microbiota Downloaded from. 2019 [cited 2020 Jan 26]. Available from: http://aem.asm.org/.
33. Dominguez-Bello MG, Costello EK, Contreras M, Magris M, Hidalgo G, Fierer N, et al. Delivery mode shapes the acquisition and structure of the initial microbiota across multiple body habitats in newborns. Proc Natl Acad Sci [Internet]. 2010 Jun 29;107(26):11971–5. Available from: http://www.pnas.org/cgi/doi/10.1073/pnas.1002601107.
34. de Steenhuijsen Piters WAA, Sanders EAM, Bogaert D. The role of the local microbial ecosystem in respiratory health and disease, vol. 370: Philosophical Transactions of the Royal Society B: Biological Sciences Royal Society of London; 2015.
35. Biesbroek G, Tsivtsivadze E, Sanders EAM, Montijn R, Veenhoven RH, Keijser BJF, et al. Early respiratory microbiota composition determines bacterial succession patterns and respiratory health in children. Am J Respir Crit Care Med. 2014;190(11):1283–92.
36. Whelan FJ, Verschoor CP, Stearns JC, Rossi L, Luinstra K, Loeb M, et al. The loss of topography in the microbial communities of the upper respiratory tract in the elderly. Ann Am Thorac Soc [Internet]. 2014 May;11(4):513–21. Available from: http://www.ncbi.nlm.nih.gov/pubmed/24601676.
37. de Steenhuijsen Piters WAA, Huijskens EGW, Wyllie AL, Biesbroek G, van den Bergh MR, Veenhoven RH, et al. Dysbiosis of upper respiratory tract microbiota in elderly pneumonia patients. ISME J [Internet]. 2016 Jan;10(1):97–108. Available from: http://www.ncbi.nlm.nih.gov/pubmed/26151645.
38. Camarinha-Silva A, Jáuregui R, Chaves-Moreno D, Oxley APA, Schaumburg F, Becker K, et al. Comparing the anterior nare bacterial community of two discrete human populations using Illumina amplicon sequencing. Environ Microbiol. 2014;16(9):2939–52.

39. Voorhies A, Ott C, Mehta S, DP-S, 2019 undefined. Study of the impact of long-duration space missions at the International Space Station on the astronaut microbiome. ncbi.nlm.nih. gov [Internet]. [cited 2020 Jan 2]. Available from: https://www.ncbi.nlm.nih.gov/pmc/articles/ PMC6616552/.
40. Abreu NA, Nagalingam NA, Song Y, Roediger FC, Pletcher SD, Goldberg AN, et al. Sinus microbiome diversity depletion and Corynebacterium tuberculostearicum enrichment mediates rhinosinusitis. Sci Transl Med. 2012;4(151).
41. Gevers D, Kugathasan S, Denson LA, Vázquez-Baeza Y, Van Treuren W, Ren B, et al. The treatment-naive microbiome in new-onset Crohn's disease. Cell Host Microbe. 2014;15(3):382–92.
42. Hartstra AV, Bouter KEC, Bäckhed F, Nieuwdorp M. Insights into the role of the microbiome in obesity and type 2 diabetes, vol. 38: Diabetes Care. American Diabetes Association Inc; 2015. p. 159–65.
43. Petersen C, Round JL. Defining dysbiosis and its influence on host immunity and disease, vol. 16: Cellular Microbiology. Blackwell Publishing Ltd; 2014. p. 1024–33.
44. Hoggard M, Waldvogel-Thurlow S, Zoing M, Chang K, Radcliff FJ, Mackenzie BW, et al. Inflammatory endotypes and microbial associations in chronic rhinosinusitis. Front Immunol. 2018;9(SEP).
45. Psaltis A, reports PW-C allergy and asthma, 2017 undefined. Therapy of sinonasal microbiome in CRS: a critical approach. Springer [Internet]. [cited 2020 Jan 2]. Available from: https://link. springer.com/article/10.1007/s11882-017-0726-x.
46. Shilts MH, Rosas-Salazar C, Tovchigrechko A, Larkin EK, Torralba M, Akopov A, et al. Minimally invasive sampling method identifies differences in taxonomic richness of nasal microbiomes in Young infants associated with mode of delivery. Microb Ecol. 2016;71(1):233–42.
47. Stearns JC, Davidson CJ, Mckeon S, Whelan FJ, Fontes ME, Schryvers AB, et al. Culture and molecular-based profiles show shifts in bacterial communities of the upper respiratory tract that occur with age. ISME J. 2015;9(5):1246–59.
48. Rosati MG, Peters AT. Relationships among allergic rhinitis, asthma, and chronic rhinosinusitis. Am J Rhinol Allergy. 2016;30(1):44–7.
49. Baroody FM, Mucha SM, deTineo M, Naclerio RM. Nasal challenge with allergen leads to maxillary sinus inflammation. J Allergy Clin Immunol. 2008;121(5)
50. Lam K, Schleimer R, Kern RC. The etiology and Pathogenesis of chronic Rhinosinusitis: a review of current hypotheses. Curr Allergy Asthma Rep Current Medicine Group LLC. 2015;15(1).
51. Fireman P. Symposium: understanding asthma pathophysiology. Allergy Asthma Proc. 2003;24(2):79–83.
52. Wagner Mackenzie B, Waite DW, Hoggard M, Douglas RG, Taylor MW, Biswas K. Bacterial community collapse: a meta-analysis of the sinonasal microbiota in chronic rhinosinusitis. Environ Microbiol [Internet]. 2017 [cited 2020 Jan 30];19(1):381–92. Available from: http:// www.ncbi.nlm.nih.gov/pubmed/27902866.
53. Lal D, Keim P, Delisle J, Barker B, Rank MA, Chia N, et al. Mapping and comparing bacterial microbiota in the sinonasal cavity of healthy, allergic rhinitis, and chronic rhinosinusitis subjects. Int Forum Allergy Rhinol. 2017;7(6):561–9.
54. Boase S, Foreman A, Cleland E, Tan L, Melton-Kreft R, Pant H, et al. The microbiome of chronic rhinosinusitis: culture, molecular diagnostics and biofilm detection. BMC Infect Dis. 2013;13(1).
55. Cope EK, Goldberg AN, Pletcher SD, Lynch S V. Compositionally and functionally distinct sinus microbiota in chronic rhinosinusitis patients have immunological and clinically divergent consequences. Microbiome [Internet]. 2017 Dec 12 [cited 2020 Jan 2];5(1):53. Available from: http://microbiomejournal.biomedcentral.com/articles/10.1186/s40168-017-0266-6.
56. Pletcher SD, Goldberg AN, Cope EK. Loss of microbial niche specificity between the upper and lower Airways in Patients with Cystic Fibrosis. Laryngoscope. 2019;129(3):544–50.

57. Sokolowska M, Frei R, Lunjani N, Akdis CA, O'Mahony L. Microbiome and asthma. Asthma Res Pract [Internet]. 2018 Dec 5 [cited 2020 Jan 30];4(1):1. Available from: https://asthmarp. biomedcentral.com/articles/10.1186/s40733-017-0037-y.

58. Huang YJ, Nariya S, Harris JM, Lynch SV, Choy DF, Arron JR, et al. The airway microbiome in patients with severe asthma: associations with disease features and severity. J Allergy Clin Immunol. 2015;136(4):874–84.

59. Huang YJ, Nelson CE, Brodie EL, Desantis TZ, Baek MS, Liu J, et al. Airway microbiota and bronchial hyperresponsiveness in patients with suboptimally controlled asthma. J Allergy Clin Immunol. 2011;127(2).

60. Frayman KB, Armstrong DS, Grimwood K, Ranganathan SC. The airway microbiota in early cystic fibrosis lung disease. Pediatr Pulmonol. 2017;52(11):1384–404.

61. Mika M, Korten I, Qi W, Regamey N, Frey U, Casaulta C, et al. The nasal microbiota in infants with cystic fibrosis in the first year of life: a prospective cohort study. Lancet Respir Med [Internet]. 2016 Aug;4(8):627–35. Available from: https://linkinghub.elsevier.com/retrieve/pii/ S2213260016300819.

62. Prevaes SMPJ, De Winter-De Groot KM, Janssens HM, De Steenhuijsen Piters WAA, Tramper-Stranders GA, Wyllie AL, et al. Development of the nasopharyngeal microbiota in infants with cystic fibrosis. Am J Respir Crit Care Med 2016;193(5):504–515.

63. Renwick J, McNally P, John B, DeSantis T, Linnane B, Murphy P. The microbial community of the cystic fibrosis airway is disrupted in early life. PLoS One. 2014;9(12).

64. Harris JK, De Groote MA, Sagel SD, Zemanick ET, Kapsner R, Penvari C, et al. Molecular identification of bacteria in bronchoalveolar lavage fluid from children with cystic fibrosis. Proc Natl Acad Sci [Internet]. 2007 Dec 18;104(51):20529–33. Available from: http://www. pnas.org/cgi/doi/10.1073/pnas.0709804104.

65. Cox MJ, Allgaier M, Taylor B, Baek MS, Huang YJ, Daly RA, et al. Airway microbiota and pathogen abundance in age-stratified cystic fibrosis patients. PLoS One. 2010;5(6)

66. Quinn RA, Lim YW, Maughan H, Conrad D, Rohwer F, Whiteson KL. Biogeochemical forces shape the composition and physiology of polymicrobial communities in the cystic fibrosis lung. MBio. 2014;5(2).

67. Coburn B, Wang PW, Diaz Caballero J, Clark ST, Brahma V, Donaldson S, et al. Lung microbiota across age and disease stage in cystic fibrosis. Sci Rep. 2015;5.

68. Delhaes L, Monchy S, Fréalle E, Hubans C, Salleron J, Leroy S, et al. The airway microbiota in cystic fibrosis: a complex fungal and bacterial community-implications for therapeutic management. PLoS One. 2012;7(4).

69. Filkins LM, Hampton TH, Gifford AH, Gross MJ, Hogan DA, Sogin ML, et al. Prevalence of streptococci and increased polymicrobial diversity associated with cystic fibrosis patient stability. J Bacteriol. 2012;194(17):4709–17.

70. Stressmann FA, Rogers GB, Van Der Gast CJ, Marsh P, Vermeer LS, Carroll MP, et al. Long-term cultivation-independent microbial diversity analysis demonstrates that bacterial communities infecting the adult cystic fibrosis lung show stability and resilience. Thorax. 2012;67(10):867–73.

71. Zemanick ET, Wagner BD, Robertson CE, Stevens MJ, Szefler SJ, Accurso FJ, et al. Assessment of airway microbiota and inflammation in cystic fibrosis using multiple sampling methods. Ann Am Thorac Soc [Internet]. 2015 Feb [cited 2020 Jan 31];12(2):221–9. Available from: http://www.atsjournals.org/doi/10.1513/AnnalsATS.201407-310OC.

72. Fujimura KE, Lynch SV. Microbiota in allergy and asthma and the emerging relationship with the gut microbiome. Cell Host Microbe Cell Press. 2015;17:592–602.

73. Markle JGM, Frank DN, Mortin-Toth S, Robertson CE, Feazel LM, Rolle-Kampczyk U, et al. Sex Differences in the Gut Microbiome Drive Hormone-Dependent Regulation of Autoimmunity [Internet]. [cited 2020 Jan 31]. Available from: http://science.sciencemag.org/.

74. Khosravi A, Mazmanian SK. Disruption of the gut microbiome as a risk factor for microbial infections. Curr Opin Microbiol. 2013;16:221–7.

75. Kalliomäki M, Kirjavainen P, Eerola E, Kero P, Salminen S, Isolauri E. Distinct patterns of neonatal gut microflora in infants in whom atopy was and was not developing. J Allergy Clin Immunol. 2001;107(1):129–34.
76. Penders J, Stobberingh EE, Thijs C, Adams H, Vink C, van Ree R, et al. Molecular fingerprinting of the intestinal microbiota of infants in whom atopic eczema was or was not developing. Clin Exp Allergy [Internet]. 2006 Dec [cited 2020 Jan 31];36(12):1602–8. Available from: http://doi.wiley.com/10.1111/j.1365-2222.2006.02599.x.
77. Fujimura KE, Demoor T, Rauch M, Faruqi AA, Jang S, Johnson CC, et al. House dust exposure mediates gut microbiome Lactobacillus enrichment and airway immune defense against allergens and virus infection. Proc Natl Acad Sci U S A. 2014;111(2):805–10.
78. Burke DG, Fouhy F, Harrison MJ, Rea MC, Cotter PD, O'sullivan O, et al. The altered gut microbiota in adults with cystic fibrosis. [cited 2020 Jan 31]. Available from: http://pyro.cme.msu.edu/.
79. Madan JC, Koestler DC, Stanton BA, Davidson L, Moulton LA, Housman ML, et al. Serial analysis of the gut and respiratory microbiome in cystic fibrosis in infancy: interaction between intestinal and respiratory tracts and impact of nutritional exposures. 2012 [cited 2020 Jan 31]. Available from: http://mbio.asm.org/.
80. Jervis Bardy J, Psaltis AJ. Next generation sequencing and the microbiome of chronic Rhinosinusitis: a primer for clinicians and review of current research, its limitations, and future Directions. Ann Otol Rhinol Laryngol [Internet]. 2016 Aug [cited 2020 Jan 2];125(8):613–21. Available from: http://www.ncbi.nlm.nih.gov/pubmed/27056556.
81. Vandelaar LJ, Hanson B, Marino M, Yao WC, Luong AU, Arias CA, et al. Analysis of Sinonasal microbiota in exacerbations of chronic Rhinosinusitis subgroups. OTO Open. 2019;3(3):2473974X1987510.
82. Haider AA, Marino MJ, Yao WC, Citardi MJ, Luong AU. The potential of high-throughput DNA sequencing of the paranasal sinus microbiome in diagnosing odontogenic sinusitis. Otolaryngol Head Neck Surg [Internet]. 2019 Dec [cited 2020 Jan 2];161(6):1043–7. Available from: http://www.ncbi.nlm.nih.gov/pubmed/31382814.
83. Rapoport SK, Smith AJ, Bergman M, Scriven KA, Brook I, Mikula SK. Determining the utility of standard hospital microbiology testing: comparing standard microbiology cultures with DNA sequence analysis in patients with chronic sinusitis. World J Otorhinolaryngol - Head Neck Surg. 2019;5(2):82–7.
84. Shen NT, Leff JA, Schneider Y, Crawford CV, Maw A, Bosworth B, et al. Cost-effectiveness analysis of probiotic use to prevent Clostridium difficile infection in hospitalized adults receiving antibiotics. Open Forum Infect Dis. 2017;4(3).
85. De Vrese M, Winkler P, Rautenberg P, Vaccine TH-, 2006 undefined. Probiotic bacteria reduced duration and severity but not the incidence of common cold episodes in a double blind, randomized, controlled trial. Elsevier [Internet]. [cited 2019 Dec 18]. Available from: https://www.sciencedirect.com/science/article/pii/S0264410X06006414.
86. Kitz R, Martens U, Zieseniß E, Enck P, Rose MA. Probiotic E. faecalis - adjuvant therapy in children with recurrent rhinosinusitis. Cent Eur J Med. 2012;7(3):362–5.
87. Guillemard E, Tondu F, Lacoin F, Schrezenmeir J. Consumption of a fermented dairy product containing the probiotic Lactobacillus casei DN-114001 reduces the duration of respiratory infections in the elderly in a randomised controlled trial. Br J Nutr. 2010;103(1):58–68.
88. Ozen M, Kocabas Sandal G, Dinleyici EC. Probiotics for the prevention of pediatric upper respiratory tract infections: a systematic review. Expert Opin Biol Ther [Internet]. 2015 Jan 2 [cited 2020 Jan 31];15(1):9–20. Available from: http://www.tandfonline.com/doi/full/10.151 7/14712598.2015.980233.
89. Bertelsen RJ, Brantsæter AL, Magnus MC, Haugen M, Myhre R, Jacobsson B, et al. Probiotic milk consumption in pregnancy and infancy and subsequent childhood allergic diseases. J Allergy Clin Immunol. 2014;133(1)

90. Bruzzese E, Raia V, Spagnuolo MI, Volpicelli M, De Marco G, Maiuri L, et al. Effect of Lactobacillus GG supplementation on pulmonary exacerbations in patients with cystic fibrosis: a pilot study. Clin Nutr. 2007;26(3):322–8.
91. Nagalingam N, Cope E, microbiology SL-T in, 2013 undefined. Probiotic strategies for treatment of respiratory diseases. Elsevier [Internet]. [cited 2019 Dec 18]. Available from: https://www.sciencedirect.com/science/article/pii/S0966842X13000826.
92. Schwartz J, Peres A, et al. LE-A journal of, 2016 undefined. Topical probiotics as a therapeutic alternative for chronic rhinosinusitis: a preclinical proof of concept. journals.sagepub.com [Internet]. [cited 2019 Dec 18]. Available from: https://journals.sagepub.com/doi/abs/10.2500/ajra.2016.30.4372.
93. Bidossi A, De Grandi R, Toscano M, Bottagisio M, De Vecchi E, Gelardi M, et al. Probiotics Streptococcus salivarius 24SMB and Streptococcus oralis 89a interfere with biofilm formation of pathogens of the upper respiratory tract. BMC Infect Dis. 2018;18(1)
94. Spacova I, Petrova MI, Fremau A, Pollaris L, Vanoirbeek J, Ceuppens JL, et al. Intranasal administration of probiotic *Lactobacillus rhamnosus* GG prevents birch pollen-induced allergic asthma in a murine model. Allergy [Internet]. 2019 Jan 8 [cited 2020 Jan 31];74(1):100–10. Available from: https://onlinelibrary.wiley.com/doi/abs/10.1111/all.13502.
95. Psaltis AJ, Wormald PJ. Therapy of Sinonasal microbiome in CRS: a critical approach. In: Current allergy and asthma reports, vol. 17: Current Medicine Group LLC; 2017. p. 1.
96. Ramakrishnan VR, Holt J, Nelson LF, Ir D, Robertson CE, Frank DN. Determinants of the Nasal Microbiome: Pilot Study of Effects of Intranasal Medication Use. Allergy Rhinol (Providence) [Internet]. [cited 2019 Oct 31];9:2152656718789519. Available from: http://www.ncbi.nlm.nih.gov/pubmed/30128169.
97. Principi N, Esposito S. Nasal irrigation: an imprecisely defined medical procedure, vol. 14. MDPI AG: International Journal of Environmental Research and Public Health; 2017.
98. Hauser LJ, Ir D, Kingdom TT, Robertson CE, Frank DN, Ramakrishnan VR. Investigation of bacterial repopulation after sinus surgery and perioperative antibiotics. Int Forum Allergy Rhinol [Internet]. 2016 Jan [cited 2020 Jan 2];6(1):34–40. Available from: http://doi.wiley.com/10.1002/alr.21630.
99. Kim AS, Willis AL, Laubitz D, Sharma S, Song BH, Chiu AG, et al. The effect of maxillary sinus antrostomy size on the sinus microbiome. Int Forum Allergy Rhinol [Internet]. 2019 [cited 2019 Oct 31];9(1):30–8. Available from: http://www.ncbi.nlm.nih.gov/pubmed/30358937.

Chapter 2
Allergic Rhinitis and Chronic Rhinosinusitis

Samuel N. Helman, Thomas S. Edwards, John M. DelGaudio, and Sarah K. Wise

Key Concepts
- Allergic rhinitis (AR) is an IgE-mediated inflammatory process with a life-time prevalence of 11–33% in the United States.
- Several subtypes of CRS are associated with AR, including allergic fungal rhinosinusitis and central compartment atopic disease.
- Allergy-mediated inflammation may represent a primary driver of CRS inflammation.

Allergic rhinitis (AR) is an inflammatory condition of the nasal cavity which is induced by exposure to aeroallergens and leads to three cardinal symptoms: sneezing, nasal obstruction, and rhinorrhea [1]. AR is mediated by immunoglobulin E (IgE) pathways and downstream effectors. After initial exposure to an aeroallergen, antigen-presenting cells (APCs) process the allergen and activate Th2 (CD4$^+$) lymphocytes. These Th2 cells induce B-cells to differentiate into plasma cells and begin production of specific IgE (sIgE) to these allergens. These sIgE molecules bind to the surface of mast cells, priming them. Re-exposure to the allergen leads to early- and late-phase inflammatory responses [1, 2]. The early-phase response involves IgE molecules on the surface of mast cells cross-linking by the re-exposed allergen leading to a release of histamine, proteases, and cytokines. Nasal itching, nasal obstruction, and rhinorrhea occur within minutes of exposure and are early clinical manifestations of AR. The late-phase response begins 4 to 8 hours after exposure

S. N. Helman · T. S. Edwards · J. M. DelGaudio · S. K. Wise (✉)
Department of Otolaryngology – Head and Neck Surgery, Emory University, Atlanta, GA, USA
e-mail: skmille@emory.edu

© Springer Nature Switzerland AG 2020
D. A. Gudis, R. J. Schlosser (eds.), *The Unified Airway*,
https://doi.org/10.1007/978-3-030-50330-7_2

and leads to worsened nasal obstruction with potential hyposmia. This phase is driven by an array of cell types (eosinophils, basophils, monocytes, macrophages, and lymphocytes) that release additional proinflammatory substances [1, 2].

AR is the most common chronic childhood disease and the fifth most common chronic disease overall in the USA [3]. AR has an estimated lifetime prevalence of 11–33% in the USA [1] and 10–40% worldwide [4, 5]. AR represents a significant cost to society, accounting for $4.5 billion in direct care and $3.4 billion in indirect costs such as work or school absenteeism for a total cost of $5.9–7.9 billion per annum [5, 6].

Similar to AR, chronic rhinosinusitis (CRS) is an inflammatory disorder of the nasal cavity and sinuses. This condition is defined as 12 weeks of sinonasal inflammation, characterized by nasal obstruction, mucoid anterior or posterior nasal drainage, facial pain/pressure/fullness, and decreased sense of smell. These symptoms must be accompanied by objective findings of inflammation on nasal endoscopy (purulence, polyps, or edema) or imaging [7]. The mechanism behind CRS is multifactorial. Generally speaking, local tissue aberrations such as epithelial tissue hypersensitivity, disruptions of innate immunity, epithelial barrier and mucociliary dysfunction, the presence of bacterial colonization and biofilm, genetic and environmental factors, and other potential etiologies may all play a role in CRS pathogenesis. These categories paint the disease process in broad strokes however, and recent data suggests that there are discrete endotypes within these categories that better refine treatment and management strategies [8]. Nonetheless, inflammation serves as a common denominator for these seemingly disparate causes of CRS.

Approximately 11.1 million adults, or 4.9% of the population of the USA, have a diagnosis of CRS. The estimated direct cost from this disease is $8.6 billion per year with the indirect cost estimated at $12.8 billion per year. While there is geographic variation, in North American and European countries, the prevalence of CRS ranges from 4.5% to 12% [9, 10].

Given that AR and CRS both demonstrate inflammation in the sinonasal region, it is reasonable to consider that allergy may produce or exacerbate CRS. However, data is conflicting when analyzing this relationship, particularly when patients are placed into broad phenotypic categories such as CRS with or without nasal polyposis [11]. This chapter examines and collates data regarding the relationship between allergy and specific subtypes of CRS.

Clinical Presentation

Patient Demographics and Medical Context

AR accounts for three million physician office visits per year in the USA, where the prevalence of AR ranges from 11% to 33% of the population depending on whether physician-diagnosed or patient-reported AR is used [1, 12]. In Europe, the prevalence of AR ranges between 10% and 41% in adults [13, 14]. An even distribution is seen between men and women [15]. AR is common in children. The prevalence of AR rises during infancy, peaks in childhood and adolescence, and falls in the elderly. In a meta-analysis of over 1.4 million children from 0 to 18 years of age in the International Study of Asthma and Allergies in Childhood (ISAAC), the overall prevalence of AR was 12.66% [16].

Generally, the prevalence of AR is difficult to estimate as these measures mainly rely on reports of "hay fever," "nasal allergies," or nasal symptoms "when you did not have a cold or the flu." Another complicating factor is the incongruence of physician- or patient-reported diagnosis of AR with results of objective measures of allergen sensitivity: skin prick testing (SPT) and/or sIgE testing. Of patients who self-report AR, 23–47.3% have negative testing for allergen sensitivity [17]. While some of this discordance may be secondary to local allergic rhinitis, patients have some degree of recall bias and/or misdiagnosis when self-reporting AR. Importantly, AR is a stop on the "atopic march" from atopic dermatitis to allergic asthma [3]. Most patients with asthma have AR, and 10–40% of patients with AR have asthma [1].

CRS is estimated to have a prevalence of 10–15% [9, 10]. Similar to AR, prevalence is difficult to assess as population-based surveys do not typically differentiate between acute and chronic sinusitis. Additionally, there is even less data to allow the estimation of the prevalence of subtypes of CRS. The 2008 Global Allergy and Asthma European Network (GA²LEN) questionnaire-based survey adhered to diagnostic criteria published in the European Position Paper on Rhinosinusitis and Nasal Polyps (EPOS), thus allowing for classification as acute vs. chronic rhinosinusitis. This survey went further, and patients underwent evaluation by an otolaryngologist to confirm a diagnosis of CRS. This work, likely the strongest estimate, reported the prevalence of CRS in Europe to be 10% [18, 19]. Best estimates of the prevalence of rhinosinusitis in the USA are approximately 12% [9]. In the 2012 US National Health Interview Survey, a patient-reported survey that did not differentiate between acute and chronic sinusitis, sinusitis was more common in women (14.5% vs. 9.0%). The prevalence of sinusitis rises during young adult life, peaks in middle age, and falls in the elderly [15]. Overall, AR and CRS are widely prevalent and clinically relevant with significant impacts on quality of life and productivity and strong associations with other comorbidities.

Signs and Symptoms

CRS without nasal polyposis is characterized by 12 weeks or more of two or more symptoms of nasal discharge, nasal obstruction or congestion, facial and sinus pain or pressure, loss of smell and/or taste, *and* objective evidence of sinonasal inflammation of intranasal examination or on radiographs. CRS with nasal polyposis requires the aforementioned criteria *plus* documentation of nasal polyposis [18].

AR is distinguished by nasal or eye itchiness, nasal congestion, and sneezing, with the potential for other accompanying symptoms such as clear rhinorrhea or postnasal drip. More generally, AR is defined as inflammation of the mucosa of the nose in response to an allergen. AR may be classified as seasonal or perennial.

Seasonal AR is most frequently triggered by tree pollens, grasses, weed pollens, or mold spores. Perennial AR is mediated by dust mites, cockroaches, pet dander, or household molds [1, 3, 5]. Episodic AR can occur during exposures to allergens that an individual is not typically exposed to as part of their usual environment. AR may also be classified by severity, similar to asthma – including intermittent vs. persistent and mild/moderate/severe classifications [4]. Physical examination can demonstrate clear nasal rhinorrhea. On endoscopy, boggy and congested nasal turbinates and pale nasal mucosa can be seen. Recently described middle turbinate or central compartment polyps/polypoid edema may also be seen on endoscopy as a manifestation of the allergic nasal response (Figs. 2.1 and 2.2) [20–22]. Extranasal examination is characterized by watery eyes with edematous conjunctiva and injected sclera, allergic shiners, and a transverse nasal crease or so-called allergic salute.

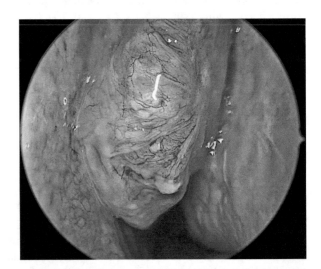

Fig. 2.1 Rigid nasal endoscopy of the left nasal cavity with large septal polyp abutting the left inferior turbinate

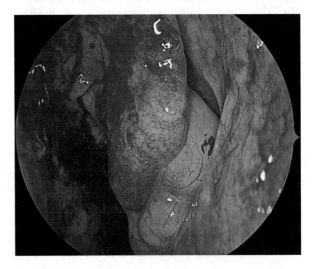

Fig. 2.2 Intraoperative nasal endoscopy of the left nasal cavity with large polyp emanating from the left middle turbinate

Similarities between AR and CRS mandate an astute and studied approach to diagnosis. The patient's history is key to distinguishing the underlying pathology. Questions should center on reported allergens, seasonal or perennial symptoms, symptoms with specific environmental exposures, symptom duration, and itchy eyes, lips, or nose as well as the patient's success with prior medical management regimens. Determining cockroach, dust mite, mold, and pet exposure is helpful as CRS is associated with perennial allergy [23]. Indeed, 56.4% of patients with CRSwNP have a perennial allergic sensitivity [24]. Chronic inflammation has many precipitants, and long-standing exposure to perennial allergens could subserve the local inflammatory milieu driving CRS.

Asthma and reactive airway disease should be a component of the history as well due to the relatively high prevalence of asthma in both AR and CRSwNP. A recent study showed the overall prevalence of asthma in CRSwNP to be 45.5%, with 100% in AERD but only 17.1% in isolated CCAD and 19% in AFRS [25]. Patients with a history of asthma, airway reactivity to aspirin or NSAIDs, and endoscopic evidence of nasal polyposis meet criteria for aspirin-exacerbated respiratory disease (AERD).

Certain CRS subtypes have specific distinguishing features that may coexist in AR and CRS. Allergic fungal rhinosinusitis (AFRS) is classically defined by Bent and Kuhn as nasal polyps with the presence of allergic mucin and fungal elements in patients with a systemic type I hypersensitivity to inhaled fungal elements [26]. AFRS can present with a diverse clinical severity from nasal obstruction and rhinitis, smell and taste loss, to marked cosmetic deformity with orbital proptosis, vision change, and intracranial sequelae [7, 27]. Patients with AFRS are typically younger and allergic/atopic with an intact immune system and present with symptoms of CRS and nasal obstruction [28]. Endoscopic evidence of nasal polyps and polypoid edema in conjunction with typical imaging features helps establish this diagnosis. Thick, allergic mucin may also be seen on nasal endoscopy in some cases of AFRS; however, mucin is not always visible on endoscopy as it may be located deep within the sinus cavities and/or obstructed by polyposis. Characteristic radiologic findings of AFRS are discussed later in this chapter.

Central compartment atopic disease (CCAD), a nasal inflammatory variant of CRSwNP that is highly associated with inhalant allergies, was first described in 2017. In this cohort, patients have endoscopic evidence of central sinonasal polyposis, mucosal edema, and/or thickening. Affected sites include the superior nasal septum and the middle and superior turbinates (Figs. 2.1 and 2.2). Imaging features demonstrate a largely central distribution of sinonasal disease with peripheral clearing laterally in the maxillary sinuses and superiorly along the ethmoid roof (Fig. 2.3) [20–22, 29]. Studies of patients with CCAD have shown allergen sensitivity in 74–100% of patients [20, 22, 29, 30]. It is thought that chronic exposure of the central compartment to inhalant allergens via nasal airflow leads to the polypoid inflammatory changes in the exposed mucosa. The presence of multifocal middle turbinate edema has a specificity of 94.7% for inhalant allergy [21]. In a recent publication, DelGaudio et al. [31] reported that approximately 90% of AERD patients had clinical AR and over 82% had endoscopic evidence of central compartment polyps.

Fig. 2.3 Coronal view of sinus computed tomography scan revealing diffuse polyps in the central compartment with peripheral clearing laterally in the maxillary sinuses and superiorly along the left ethmoid roof, indicative of CCAD

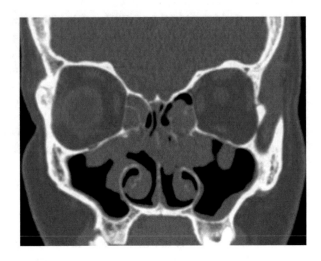

Diagnostics

The process of diagnosing AR in CRS requires thorough history taking and a focused head and neck and nasal endoscopic examination. Features noted in Sect. "Signs and Symptoms" bring about consideration of AR or CRS, with allergy testing and imaging further corroborating initial findings. This chapter uses AFRS and CCAD as archetypes of the relationship between allergy and CRS, but the astute practitioner should keep in mind several other disease entities encompassed within CRSwNP, including AERD, CRSwNP not otherwise specified (NOS), and cystic fibrosis. In the setting of unilateral polyposis, nasal tumor and inverted papilloma should be considered. Respiratory epithelial adenomatoid hamartoma (REAH) can be unilateral or bilateral and is often delimited to the upper nasal septum or co-occurs with CRSwNP [32, 33]. This section will focus on systemic allergy testing and imaging as a means of narrowing the differential diagnosis. Endoscopic findings of the AFRS and CCAD CRS subtypes were discussed in Sect. "Signs and Symptoms."

Atopy, or the triggering of an IgE-mediated response as a result of an allergen exposure, is what drives AR [11]. Skin or serum allergy testing is key modality to determine sensitivity to an allergen. It is important to note, however, that sensitivity on testing simply means that the patient is reactive to that allergen on the test. Clinical AR is present when the patient is sensitive to an allergen *and* exhibits symptoms upon exposure to the allergen. Not all patients who are sensitive will demonstrate clinical AR symptoms. Allergy skin testing for aeroallergen reactivity may be performed via skin prick, intradermal, or blended techniques. Serum in vitro testing is also an option for diagnosis of allergen sensitivity. Interestingly, while skin and in vitro allergy testing is not commonly employed simultaneously, this may prove useful in certain patients as there may be some variability between the two techniques and some sensitivities may otherwise be missed [34–36]. An in-depth discussion of allergy testing techniques is beyond the scope of this chapter. However, established protocols should be followed, with assurance of appropriate positive and negative controls, avoidance of interfering medications during skin testing, and trained personnel performing and interpreting the testing. Allergy testing should be considered in patients with allergic symptoms or endoscopic/radiologic evidence of sinonasal disease consistent with an allergic subtype.

Allergy testing is quite helpful in definitively diagnosing AR and has a key role in several CRS endotypes, including CCAD, AFRS, and AERD with CCAD features. In CCAD, for example, 100% of this cohort had positive allergy testing and clinical AR [20]. Marcus et al. [25] determined that allergy was significantly higher in AFRS (100%), CCAD (97.6%), CRSwNP with central compartment polypoid disease (97.6%), and AERD (84.6%) compared with CRSwNP not otherwise specified (56.1%). Fungal sIgE is detected by allergy testing in AFRS, and total IgE is often elevated up to 5000 IU/mL, with a mean of 600 IU/mL [27, 37]. Skin and serum testing demonstrates several possible environmental etiologies include a host of *Aspergillus* species as well as the dematiaceous fungi such as *Bipolaris, Curvularia, Alternaria*, and *Fusarium* [27].

Discord between systemic allergy testing and clinical manifestations of allergy can occur, whereby intranasal exposure to allergen can lead to local eosinophilia, histamine, and pro-inflammatory cytokine production [38–40]. While commercial testing for intranasal cytokines and inflammatory cells adds useful information to the inflammatory mosaic of AR and CRS, such testing is infrequently employed in routine clinical practice [31].

Of note, systemic allergy testing is a useful, but imperfect, technique. Indeed, 26.5% of individuals previously classified as nonatopic may have an intranasal sIgE response to allergen exposure [21, 41, 42]. This discord between systemic and local allergen responses has been well characterized and results from local allergen response at the tissue level. Local allergic rhinitis is typically diagnosed via intranasal allergen challenge, detection of sIgE in nasal secretions/tissues, or basophil activation testing – techniques which are still considered experimental in many regions.

Computed tomography (CT) has proven to be a helpful adjunct in identifying and classifying paranasal sinus disease. AFRS and CCAD have relatively consistent CT features that can be distinguished on imaging. Central compartment disease is aptly named, as there is central compartment soft tissue edema and polyposis evidence on endoscopy and CT imaging. Sinusitis can occur in these patients as a result of middle turbinate lateralization or from direct polypoid obstruction of the sinus outflow tracts (Fig. 2.3) [20]. Imaging that demonstrates central compartment hypodensity/opacity with clearing in the adjoining paranasal sinuses is associated strongly with allergy, predicting atopic disease with 90.82% specificity and a positive predictive value of 73.53% [29].

AFRS has relatively conserved findings on CT and MRI. CT demonstrates heterogeneous intrasinus densities and may have marked bony thinning of the paranasal sinus walls with remodeling and distortion of the native anatomy (Fig. 2.4). Wise et al. [43], in a review of 111 CT scans, determined that bony abnormalities were present in the ethmoid sinuses in 77% of graded patients, versus 68% of the

Fig. 2.4 Coronal view of
sinus computed
tomography scan revealing
marked distortion of native
anatomy with bony
thinning and remodeling,
indicative of AFRS

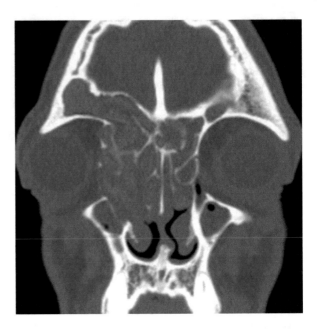

maxillary, 58% of the sphenoid, and 53% of the frontal sinuses. With magnetic resonance imaging (MRI), increased T1 signal intensity and T2 signal is variable; however, in areas of sludge or mycetoma, high protein content (25–40%) can yield low T1 signal intensity and a signal void on T2-weighted images [44].

While no pathognomonic radiologic features of allergy exist, there is nonetheless evidence of sinonasal inflammation on plain films (56.3% affected) and CT scans of allergic patients (67.5%) [45, 46]. Moreover, patients undergoing a nasal provocation test with cypress pollen have evidence of inflammation in images of their osteomeatal complexes and the ethmoid sinus [47]. Nonetheless, imaging is not recommended in AR alone and should not be routinely performed if symptoms are consistent with standard AR [3].

Medical Management

When broadly considering AR and CRS as separate entities, medical management of each of these conditions demonstrates as many similarities as differences. Where the two entities meet is in the management of chronic sinonasal inflammation. Non-pharmacologic therapies for AR include avoidance of known allergens, environmental controls such as removing pets, and use of air filtration systems, acaricides, and bed/pillow covers [1]. Identifying and treating comorbid asthma, atopic dermatitis, and otitis is a helpful adjunct when treating more severe AR. First-line therapies consist of nasal steroids and second-generation oral antihistamines for patients with sneezing and itching. Intranasal antihistamines and sublingual (SLIT) or subcutaneous immunotherapy (SCIT) are additional options [3, 48].

For the purposes of this article, the authors have elected to address the medical management of CRS as it relates to allergy-exacerbated CRS. Broadly discussing the medical management of CRS in general is beyond the scope of this chapter; however, it should be noted that currently accepted therapy for Th2-mediated CRSwNP subtypes includes high-volume nasal saline irrigations and topical intranasal corticosteroids, often in the form of off-label steroid irrigations.

Allergy has a high prevalence in AFRS (100%), CCAD (97.6%), CRSwNP and concomitant central compartment polypoid disease (84.6%), and AERD (82.6%) when compared with CRSwNP NOS (56.1%) [25, 31]. It follows that therapies directed toward allergy control should offer benefit in the CRS endotypes that have high allergy prevalence. As such, immunotherapy in the form of SLIT or SCIT may have a role in these patient groups. Nonetheless, in a review of the relationship between allergy and CRS, Marcus et al. [49] determined the evidence for immunotherapy in the management of CCAD and AFRS to be weak, despite the strong evidence supporting the association of AFRS and CCAD with allergy. As such, the decision to start SCIT or SLIT should be tailored to the individual patients and should be the product of shared decision-making in light of the available evidence [50].

Biologic therapies have had an increasing role in the management of CRSwNP, becoming especially poignant with the approval of dupilumab by the US FDA in June 2019. While no biologic therapy has been specifically tailored toward AFRS, CCAD, or AR in CRS, targeted anti-IgE may play a role in certain CRS endotypes in the future. Omalizumab, which has already entered the market for allergen-exacerbated refractory asthma and chronic urticaria, has also been studied in CRSwNP [51]. In one study, omalizumab led to a reduction in total nasal endoscopic polyp scores, and allergic patients had marked improvements in their Lund-Mackay scores compared to nonallergic peers, suggesting IgE as a target for therapeutics in CRSwNP. Gan et al. [52] studied seven patients with moderate to severe asthma as well as prior sinus surgery and in-office polypectomies. The patients were treated with omalizumab injections every 2–4 weeks, and 86% reported a reduction in sinus symptoms and improved quality of life following treatment. Patients using budesonide rinses were able to either reduce (43%) or completely discontinue therapy (14%), and no patients required subsequent surgery during the follow-up period. It is anticipated that we will see several additional targeted biologic therapies enter the market for CRSwNP, in addition to dupilumab, in the coming years.

Surgical Management

Surgical management is reserved for medically refractory cases of AFRS and CCAD and has little role in pure AR beyond inferior turbinate reduction in patients who have failed medical management [3]. While AR and CRS may coexist, the decision for surgical management is predicated on CRS symptoms and response to medical management. With this in mind, the surgery should be planned with the specific disease process in mind. It is possible that extensive endoscopic sinus surgery may expose areas of the sinus that were previously sequestered from aeroallergen. Indeed, in the unoperated sinus, inhaled radiolabeled aeroallergens are by and large retained in the nasal cavities and do not enter the sinuses [53]. It follows that after surgery the sinuses are now exposed to allergen. Therefore, medical and surgical management should go hand in hand, and concomitant immunotherapy may be a valuable adjunct to reduce the inflammation caused by inhaled aeroallergen [1].

AFRS allergic fungal mucin is a tenacious material. Histopathologic analysis demonstrates Charcot-Leyden crystals (which occur from eosinophilic degradation), eosinophil granulocytes, as well as sparse and noninvasive fungal hyphae [26]. The presence of allergic mucin is also characteristic for AFRS. Removal of obstructive mucin with surgery relieves the source of local inflammation. In AFRS, surgery involves widely opening the paranasal sinuses in a sequential fashion and removing allergic mucin and obstructing partitions [54]. Classic sinonasal anatomy may be grossly distorted by disease, and image-guided navigation is frequently used. Widely opening the sinuses of a patient with AFRS facilitates irrigations and topical therapies. It is essential to remove all inspissated mucin from the sinuses, in particular in hard-to-reach recesses of the frontal, sphenoid, and maxillary sinuses. Abandoned mucin likely serves as a nidus for inflammation and obstructs topical therapies from reaching inflamed mucosa. Indeed, AFRS has a strong association with need for revision surgery [55]. While there are no rigorous randomized controlled trials examining postoperative regimens in AFRS, maintenance steroid irrigations and considering immunotherapy are reasonable options in the management of this disease [52, 54].

In CCAD, DelGaudio et al. [20] primarily manage this cohort with maintenance intranasal corticosteroids, short courses of oral corticosteroids, and consideration of allergen immunotherapy. Patients who are refractory to this management undergo surgical therapy to debulk obstructive central compartment disease and manage the affected adjacent sinuses. The authors describe, "sculpting" the central compartment polypoid disease primarily, but advise more extensive surgical intervention to clear frontal sinus pathology, remove extensive central compartment polyps, and clear prior synechia to allow for better access for topical medications.

In AERD with CCAD, the middle turbinates may be protective for inhalant aeroallergens, and the authors suggest consideration of a conservative approach to the middle turbinates. In particular, septal polypoid disease that extends anterior to the middle turbinate should be trimmed, and septal disease should be sculpted to allow for postoperative topical irrigations. In severe disease, the authors recommend an endoscopic Lothrop procedure as a means of resecting polypoid or polyp-bearing mucosa from the upper nasal septum anterior to the middle turbinates [20]. Postoperatively, patients are treated with high-volume topical steroid rises. Allergen immunotherapy is a consideration if patients are sensitive and symptomatic to inhalant allergens. Therefore, the most appropriate treatment is multifactorial, but surgery is essential as a means of relieving sinus obstruction and allowing proper medication delivery. In this patient population, immunotherapy and aspirin sensitization should be considered.

Impact of Rhinologic Interventions

This section will address surgical outcomes in AFRS, AERD with CCAD, and CCAD. Complete surgery to remove trapped mucin and marsupialize the sinuses followed by thorough medical management is essential in AFRS, which has been demonstrated to be recidivistic [37, 50]. Schubert and Goetz [37] identified that 2 months of oral corticosteroids could extend clinical improvement for up to 12 months and more generally prolongs the time between subsequent sinus surgeries. Loftus et al. [55] determined that the overall revision rate in CRSwNP was 18.6%. In their meta-analysis, AERD and AFRS subgroups had significantly higher revision rates (27.2% and 28.7%) when compared to CRSwNP overall (18.6%). The study also illustrated that patients with comorbid asthma had significantly higher revision rates of 22.6% versus 8.0%.

Surgical intervention is common in AERD, and many are diagnosed with aspirin sensitivity at a late stage following several surgeries. In AERD with CCAD, patients had a mean of 3.8 surgeries as compared to 3.2 for AERD patients without central compartment involvement. In patients with central compartment involvement of the nasal septum, these patients had twice as many procedures than patients without septal involvement (4.2 versus 2.0, $p = 0.004$). Additionally, central compartment diseases with septal polyp involvement all have higher rates of middle turbinate resection, suggesting that the loss of the middle turbinates may allow for allergen deposition along the superior nasal septal mucosa and subsequent polypoid change [20]. The authors therefore recommend consideration of conservative management of the middle turbinate and middle turbinate sculpting when possible to preserve their protective role; however, outcome data for this recommendation should be collected in the future to determine its true benefit.

One interesting trend from the Loftus et al. [55] study was that surgery performed for CRSwNP after 2008 had significantly lower rates of surgical revision. The authors speculate that this could be the result of improved medical management, surgical technique facilitating nasal steroid irrigation, and improved postoperative surgical surveillance.

Case

A 65-year-old man presented for evaluation of chronic nasal obstruction. He noted worsening of symptoms over the past several months during the renovation of his home. He endorsed periorbital pressure and diminished sense of smell. He denied thick anterior nasal drainage but endorsed sneezing and thin rhinorrhea at times. His 22-item sinonasal outcome test (SNOT-22) [56] score was 51. Past medical history included asthma, psoriasis, and AR. His asthma was well controlled (FEV1/FVC 97% of predicted) with daily beclomethasone dipropionate and albuterol as needed. Daily acitretin and topical corticosteroids as needed were used to control his psoriasis. He was taking daily oral loratadine, topical azelastine and fluticasone, and nasal saline spray for his AR. He had undergone treatment with SCIT twice previously; the most recent SCIT treatment was over 20 years ago, and both were less than 2 years in length. He denied any sensitivity to aspirin or NSAIDs. He had previously undergone endoscopic sinus surgery a decade prior to his evaluation in our clinic. This improved his symptoms for several years although the symptoms slowly returned.

Rigid nasal endoscopy showed large, obstructive septal polyps bilaterally (Fig. 2.1). A non-contrast CT scan of the sinuses was obtained which showed diffuse polypoid tissue throughout the nasal cavity and the medial aspect of the maxillary sinuses with peripheral clearing (Fig. 2.3). Allergy testing was performed using the modified quantitative testing (MQT) method [57]. He was sensitive to numerous perennial and seasonal allergens (Table 2.1). Based on endoscopy and imaging findings, he was diagnosed with CCAD, and functional endoscopic sinus surgery was recommended.

He underwent bilateral endoscopic sinus surgery. Following removal of the septal polyps, polypoid middle turbinates were also noted (Fig. 2.2). The polypoid middle turbinates were sculpted but largely preserved. Following surgical intervention, he was started on high-volume topical budesonide as well as SLIT to reduce sinonasal inflammation. His symptoms improved significantly with a SNOT-22 score of 8 at three months postoperatively.

Table 2.1 Modified quantitative testing example

Panel A					Panel C				
Site: right upper forearm					**Site: left upper forearm**				
	P	**#5**	**#2**	**EP**		**P**	**#5**	**#2**	**EP**
1. Histamine (+ control)	7	–	–	–	1. Bahia	5	4	–	4
2. Mite, D.P.	13	–	–	6	2. English plantain	0	–	7	3
3. Mite, D.F.	13	–	–	6	3. Lamb's quarters	0	–	7	3
4. Alternaria	9	–	–	6	4. Birch	5	3	–	4
5. *Aspergillus*	13	–	–	6	5. White ash	5	4	–	4
6. Cat	13	–	–	6	6. E. Cottonwood	0	–	5	NEG
7. Dog	0	–	7	3	7. American elm	0	–	5	NEG
8. Glycerin (– control)	0	–	–	–	8. Red maple	4	4	–	4
Panel B					**Panel D**				
Site: right lower forearm					**Site: left lower forearm**				
	P	**#5**	**#2**	**EP**		**P**	**#5**	**#2**	**EP**
1. Cockroach	7	4	–	4	1. *Cladosporium*	0	–	4	NEG
2. Bermuda grass	5	4	–	4	2. *B. sorokiniana*	0	–	7	3
3. Timothy grass	0	–	5	NEG	3. *Penicillium*	0	–	5	NEG
4. Oak, white	5	4	–	4	4. Mouse	0	–	6	NEG
5. Pecan, pollen	0	–	7	3	5. Histamine (+ Conf ctrl)	7	–	–	+
6. Red cedar	0	–	5	NEG	6. Mixed feathers	0	–	7	3
7. Short ragweed	0	–	7	3	7. *Epicoccum*	0	–	7	3
8. Rough pigweed	0	–	9	3					

Allergy skin testing endpoints (EP) by this method range from 0 (negative; NEG) to 6 (maximum positive reactivity)

Conclusion

This chapter identifies and codifies the unique relationship that AR and allergy in general have with CRS. It is evident that there are certain CRS subtypes where allergy is prominent. Chronic inflammation defines CRS generally, and superimposed allergy-mediated inflammation may further drive AFRS and CCAD. Further evidence is needed to clarify the relationship between AR and specific CRS subtypes, particularly in the era of myriad advances in the medical and surgical management of previously recalcitrant diseases.

References

1. Wise SK, Lin SY, Toskala E, Orlandi RR, Akdis CA, Alt JA, et al. International Consensus Statement on Allergy and Rhinology: Allergic Rhinitis Int Forum Allergy Rhinol. 2018;8(2):108–352.
2. Rosenwasser LJ. Current understanding of the pathophysiology of allergic rhinitis. Immunol Allergy Clin N Am. 2011;31(3):433–9.
3. Seidman MD, Gurgel RK, Lin SY, Schwartz SR, Baroody FM, Bonner JR, et al. Clinical practice guideline: Allergic rhinitis. Otolaryngol Head Neck Surg. 2015;152(1 Suppl):S1–43.
4. Brozek JL, Bousquet J, Agache I, Agarwal A, Bachert C, Bosnic-Anticevich S, et al. Allergic rhinitis and its Impact on asthma (ARIA) guidelines-2016 revision. J Allergy Clin Immunol. 2017;140(4):950–8.
5. Bellanti JA, Wallerstedt DB. Allergic rhinitis update: epidemiology and natural history. Allergy Asthma Proc. 2000;21(6):367–70.
6. Emanuel IA, Parker MJ, Traub O. Undertreatment of allergy: exploring the utility of sublingual immunotherapy. Otolaryngol Head Neck Surg. 2009;140(5):615–21.
7. Orlandi RR, Kingdom TT, Hwang PH, Smith TL, Alt JA, Baroody FM, et al. International consensus statement on allergy and rhinology: rhinosinusitis Int Forum Allergy Rhinol. 2016;6(Suppl 1):S22–209.
8. Gurrola J 2nd, Borish L. Chronic rhinosinusitis: Endotypes, biomarkers, and treatment response. J Allergy Clin Immunol. 2017;140(6):1499–508.
9. DeConde AS, Soler ZM. Chronic rhinosinusitis: epidemiology and burden of disease. Am J Rhinol Allergy. 2016;30(2):134–9.
10. Bhattacharyya N, Villeneuve S, Joish VN, Amand C, Mannent L, Amin N, et al. Cost burden and resource utilization in patients with chronic rhinosinusitis and nasal polyps. Laryngoscope. 2019;129(9):1969–75.
11. Wilson KF, McMains KC, Orlandi RR. The association between allergy and chronic rhinosinusitis with and without nasal polyps: an evidence-based review with recommendations. Int Forum Allergy Rhinol. 2014;4(2):93–103.
12. Mattos JL, Woodard CR, Payne SC. Trends in common rhinologic illnesses: analysis of U.S. healthcare surveys 1995-2007. Int Forum Allergy Rhinol. 2011;1(1):3–12.
13. Variations in the prevalence of respiratory symptoms, self-reported asthma attacks, and use of asthma medication in the European Community Respiratory Health Survey (ECRHS). Eur Respir J. 1996;9(4):687–95.
14. Jarvis D, Newson R, Lotvall J, Hastan D, Tomassen P, Keil T, et al. Asthma in adults and its association with chronic rhinosinusitis: the GA2LEN survey in Europe. Allergy. 2012;67(1):91–8.
15. Blackwell DL, Lucas JW, Clarke TC. Summary health statistics for U.S. adults: national health interview survey, 2012. Vital Health Stat 10. 2014;(260):1–161.

16. Pols DH, Wartna JB, van Alphen EI, Moed H, Rasenberg N, Bindels PJ, et al. Interrelationships between atopic disorders in children: a meta-analysis based on ISAAC questionnaires. PLoS One. 2015;10(7):e0131869.
17. Mims JW. Epidemiology of allergic rhinitis. Int Forum Allergy Rhinol. 2014;4(Suppl 2):S18–20.
18. Fokkens WJ, Lund VJ, Mullol J, Bachert C, Alobid I, Baroody F, et al. EPOS 2012: European position paper on rhinosinusitis and nasal polyps 2012. A summary for otorhinolaryngologists. Rhinology. 2012;50(1):1–12.
19. Hastan D, Fokkens WJ, Bachert C, Newson RB, Bislimovska J, Bockelbrink A, et al. Chronic rhinosinusitis in Europe--an underestimated disease. A GA(2)LEN study. Allergy. 2011;66(9):1216–23.
20. DelGaudio JM, Loftus PA, Hamizan AW, Harvey RJ, Wise SK. Central compartment atopic disease. Am J Rhinol Allergy. 2017;31(4):228–34.
21. Hamizan AW, Christensen JM, Ebenzer J, Oakley G, Tattersall J, Sacks R, et al. Middle turbinate edema as a diagnostic marker of inhalant allergy. Int Forum Allergy Rhinol. 2017;7(1):37–42.
22. White LJ, Rotella MR, DelGaudio JM. Polypoid changes of the middle turbinate as an indicator of atopic disease. Int Forum Allergy Rhinol. 2014;4(5):376–80.
23. Gutman M, Torres A, Keen KJ, Houser SM. Prevalence of allergy in patients with chronic rhinosinusitis. Otolaryngol Head Neck Surg. 2004;130(5):545–52.
24. Houser SM, Keen KJ. The role of allergy and smoking in chronic rhinosinusitis and polyposis. Laryngoscope. 2008;118(9):1521–7.
25. Marcus S, Schertzer J, Roland LT, Wise SK, Levy JM, DelGaudio JM. Central compartment atopic disease: prevalence of allergy and asthma compared with other subtypes of chronic rhinosinusitis with nasal polyps. Int Forum Allergy Rhinol. 2020;10(2):183–9.
26. Bent JP 3rd, Kuhn FA. Diagnosis of allergic fungal sinusitis. Otolaryngol Head Neck Surg. 1994;111(5):580–8.
27. Raz E, Win W, Hagiwara M, Lui YW, Cohen B, Fatterpekar GM. Fungal Sinusitis. Neuroimaging Clin N Am. 2015;25(4):569–76.
28. Glass D, Amedee RG. Allergic fungal rhinosinusitis: a review. Ochsner J. 2011;11(3):271–5.
29. Hamizan AW, Loftus PA, Alvarado R, Ho J, Kalish L, Sacks R, et al. Allergic phenotype of chronic rhinosinusitis based on radiologic pattern of disease. Laryngoscope. 2018;128(9):2015–21.
30. Brunner JP, Jawad BA, McCoul ED. Polypoid change of the middle turbinate and paranasal sinus polyposis are distinct entities. Otolaryngol Head Neck Surg. 2017;157(3):519–23.
31. DelGaudio JM, Levy JM, Wise SK. Central compartment involvement in aspirin-exacerbated respiratory disease: the role of allergy and previous sinus surgery. Int Forum Allergy Rhinol. 2019;9(9):1017–22.
32. Mortuaire G, Pasquesoone X, Leroy X, Chevalier D. Respiratory epithelial adenomatoid hamartomas of the sinonasal tract. Eur Arch Otorhinolaryngol. 2007;264(4):451–3.
33. Nguyen DT, Jankowski R, Bey A, Gauchotte G, Casse JM, Gondim Teixeira PA, et al. Respiratory epithelial Adenomatoid hamartoma is frequent in olfactory cleft after nasalization. Laryngoscope. 2019; https://doi.org/10.1002/lary.28298.
34. de Vos G. Skin testing versus serum-specific IgE testing: which is better for diagnosing aeroallergen sensitization and predicting clinical allergy? Curr Allergy Asthma Rep. 2014;14(5):430.
35. Tan BK, Zirkle W, Chandra RK, Lin D, Conley DB, Peters AT, et al. Atopic profile of patients failing medical therapy for chronic rhinosinusitis. Int Forum Allergy Rhinol. 2011;1(2):88–94.
36. Munoz del Castillo F, Jurado-Ramos A, Fernandez-Conde BL, Soler R, Barasona MJ, Cantillo E, et al. Allergenic profile of nasal polyposis. J Investig Allergol Clin Immunol. 2009;19(2):110–6.
37. Schubert MS, Goetz DW. Evaluation and treatment of allergic fungal sinusitis. I. Demographics and diagnosis. J Allergy Clin Immunol. 1998;102(3):387–94.
38. Baroody FM, Mucha SM, Detineo M, Naclerio RM. Nasal challenge with allergen leads to maxillary sinus inflammation. J Allergy Clin Immunol. 2008;121(5):1126–32 e7.

39. Bachert C, Gevaert P, Holtappels G, Johansson SG, van Cauwenberge P. Total and specific IgE in nasal polyps is related to local eosinophilic inflammation. J Allergy Clin Immunol. 2001;107(4):607–14.
40. Mygind N, Dahl R, Bachert C. Nasal polyposis, eosinophil dominated inflammation, and allergy. Thorax. 2000;55(Suppl 2):S79–83.
41. Settipane RA, Kaliner MA. Chapter 14: nonallergic rhinitis. Am J Rhinol Allergy. 2013;27(3):48–51.
42. Rondon C, Campo P, Togias A, Fokkens WJ, Durham SR, Powe DG, et al. Local allergic rhinitis: concept, pathophysiology, and management. J Allergy Clin Immunol. 2012;129(6):1460–7.
43. Wise SK, Rogers GA, Ghegan MD, Harvey RJ, Delgaudio JM, Schlosser RJ. Radiologic staging system for allergic fungal rhinosinusitis (AFRS). Otolaryngol Head Neck Surg. 2009;140(5):735–40.
44. Manning SC, Merkel M, Kriesel K, Vuitch F, Marple B. Computed tomography and magnetic resonance diagnosis of allergic fungal sinusitis. Laryngoscope. 1997;107(2):170–6.
45. Kirtsreesakul V, Ruttanaphol S. The relationship between allergy and rhinosinusitis. Rhinology. 2008;46(3):204–8.
46. Berrettini S, Carabelli A, Sellari-Franceschini S, Bruschini L, Abruzzese A, Quartieri F, et al. Perennial allergic rhinitis and chronic sinusitis: correlation with rhinologic risk factors. Allergy. 1999;54(3):242–8.
47. Piette V, Bousquet C, Kvedariene V, Dhivert-Donnadieu H, Crampette L, Senac JP, et al. Sinus CT scans and mediator release in nasal secretions after nasal challenge with cypress pollens. Allergy. 2004;59(8):863–8.
48. Dykewicz MS, Wallace DV, Baroody F, Bernstein J, Craig T, Finegold I, et al. Treatment of seasonal allergic rhinitis: an evidence-based focused 2017 guideline update. Ann Allergy Asthma Immunol. 2017;119(6):489–511 e41.
49. Marcus S, Roland LT, DelGaudio JM, Wise SK. The relationship between allergy and chronic rhinosinusitis. Laryngoscope Investig Otolaryngol. 2019;4(1):13–7.
50. Schubert MS. Allergic fungal sinusitis. Otolaryngol Clin N Am. 2004;37(2):301–26.
51. Evans MO 2nd, Coop CA. Novel treatment of allergic fungal sinusitis using omalizumab. Allergy Rhinol (Providence). 2014;5(3):172–4.
52. Gan EC, Thamboo A, Rudmik L, Hwang PH, Ferguson BJ, Javer AR. Medical management of allergic fungal rhinosinusitis following endoscopic sinus surgery: an evidence-based review and recommendations. Int Forum Allergy Rhinol. 2014;4(9):702–15.
53. Adkins TN, Goodgold HM, Hendershott L, Slavin RG. Does inhaled pollen enter the sinus cavities? Ann Allergy Asthma Immunol. 1998;81(2):181–4.
54. Manning SC, Vuitch F, Weinberg AG, Brown OE. Allergic aspergillosis: a newly recognized form of sinusitis in the pediatric population. Laryngoscope. 1989;99(7). Pt 1:681–5.
55. Loftus CA, Soler ZM, Koochakzadeh S, Desiato VM, Yoo F, Nguyen SA, et al. Revision surgery rates in chronic rhinosinusitis with nasal polyps: meta-analysis of risk factors. Int Forum Allergy Rhinol. 2020;10(2):199–207.
56. Hopkins C, Gillett S, Slack R, Lund VJ, Browne JP. Psychometric validity of the 22-item Sinonasal outcome test. Clin Otolaryngol. 2009;34(5):447–54.
57. Marple BF, Mabry RL. Quantitative skin testing for allergy: IDT and MQT. New York: Thieme Medical Publishers; 2006. p. xiv,113.

Chapter 3
Adenoid Disease and Pediatric Chronic Rhinosinusitis

Jarret Foster, Ryan Belcher, Brittany Lipscomb, and Frank W. Virgin

> **Key Concepts**
> - The adenoids play a significant role in the pathophysiology of pediatric CRS.
> - Adenoidectomy with or without sinus surgery has a critical role in the surgical management of pediatric CRS.

Rhinosinusitis is a common disorder involving inflammation of the sinus and nasal mucosa. Typically, it is classified by the duration of symptoms: acute (less than one month), subacute (one to three months), and chronic (greater than three months) [1]. Pediatric chronic rhinosinusitis (PCRS) is defined by at least 90 continuous days of

J. Foster
University of South Carolina School of Medicine, Columbia, SC, USA

Surgical Outcomes Center for Kids (SOCKs), Vanderbilt University Medical Center, Nashville, TN, USA

R. Belcher · F. W. Virgin (✉)
Surgical Outcomes Center for Kids (SOCKs), Vanderbilt University Medical Center, Nashville, TN, USA

Department of Otolaryngology-Head & Neck Surgery, Vanderbilt University Medical Center, Nashville, TN, USA

Monroe Carell Jr. Children's Hospital at Vanderbilt, Nashville, TN, USA
e-mail: frank.w.virgin@vumc.org

B. Lipscomb
Surgical Outcomes Center for Kids (SOCKs), Vanderbilt University Medical Center, Nashville, TN, USA

Department of Otolaryngology-Head & Neck Surgery, Vanderbilt University Medical Center, Nashville, TN, USA

© Springer Nature Switzerland AG 2020
D. A. Gudis, R. J. Schlosser (eds.), *The Unified Airway*,
https://doi.org/10.1007/978-3-030-50330-7_3

any two of the following symptoms: purulent rhinorrhea, nasal obstruction, facial pressure and pain, and cough, with corresponding endoscopic or CT findings in a patient aged 18 years or younger [2]. The condition represents a significant outpatient clinic burden in pediatric ambulatory care centers nationwide, being diagnosed in 2.1% of all visits annually [3].

While the pathogenesis of adult and pediatric chronic rhinosinusitis shares many common features, the presence of adenoids is a primary distinction in the pathogenesis of PCRS. Adenoids have been shown to have a significant impact on the development of PCRS in children aged 12 years and younger [2, 4]. Adenoid contribution to pathogenesis occurs primarily through the following mechanisms: serving as a bacterial reservoir, posterior nasal obstruction, the presence of biofilms, and effects on secretory IgA.

The adenoids serve as a bacterial reservoir leading to microbiological colonization and chronic inflammation of the upper airway. These inflammatory changes may cause metaplastic changes to the nasal mucosa's ciliated epithelium [5]. These changes affect mucociliary clearance of the sinuses leading to poor clearance of sinus mucus and obstruction of sinus outflow tracks [6]. Adenoid hypertrophy can also significantly contribute to posterior nasal obstruction and impaired mucociliary clearance. The increased size of the adenoids contributes to mucus retention within the nasal cavity and leads to further inflammation and potential bacterial infection [5, 7]. While impaired mucociliary clearance can be due to adenoid involvement, it may also be due to an underlying genetic disorder. Patients with primary ciliary dyskinesia or cystic fibrosis will be more prone to PCRS due to their inherent mucociliary clearance dysfunction. While cystic fibrosis patients have a nearly 100% prevalence of PCRS on CT, many of them are relatively asymptomatic [8–11]. Patients with primary ciliary dyskinesia have a prevalence of PCRS reported to range from 11% to 71% [12, 13].

Biofilms and reduced secretory IgA are also associated with adenoid contributions to PCRS [14, 15]. Biofilms have been identified on the tonsils, adenoids, and sinus mucosa. Studies have demonstrated that biofilm formation on adenoid tissue is significantly more common in patients undergoing adenoidectomy for PCRS than in patients undergoing adenoidectomy for obstructive sleep apnea without PCRS. Biofilm formation can decrease the effectiveness of antimicrobial therapy [7, 16]. Patients with PCRS have also been shown to have lower levels of secretory IgA coating their adenoid epithelium. This enhances the colonization of the upper respiratory tract with bacteria and results in chronic inflammation [7, 15].

Clinical Presentation

PCRS may present insidiously with nonspecific symptoms over years to months, or it may present acutely as a nonspecific upper respiratory infection or sinusitis that fails to resolve. There are four cardinal symptoms associated with PCRS [17]: anterior or posterior nasal mucopurulent drainage; nasal obstruction; facial pain, pressure, or fullness; and cough.

Routine physical exam findings may include evidence of rhinorrhea, edema and erythema of the nasal mucosa, or polyps in the nasal cavity. Patients with significant adenoid involvement may present with "adenoid facies" represented by excessive mouth breathing, allergic shiners, and drooling.

The imaging study of choice for chronic rhinosinusitis is computed tomography (CT), specifically non-contrasted CT with axial, coronal, and sagittal views. However, in children, CT is generally reserved for patients who have failed medical therapy or adenoidectomy to minimize radiation exposure [18]. MRI can be used as well but has inferior resolution of bony anatomy and may require sedation or anesthesia to obtain. MRI may be preferred in patients when there is concern for orbital or intracranial extension [19–21].

Nasal endoscopy is an essential component of the evaluation for PCRS. It allows for direct visualization of the sinus drainage pathways and of the adenoid pad. Endoscopy also rules out other diagnoses such as choanal atresia, neoplasm or foreign body, and bacterial cultures if indicated. Anterior rhinoscopy is limited in its capacity to diagnose PCRS and to assess for adenoid hypertrophy.

Plain film radiographs have limited sensitivity and specificity for the diagnosis of PCRS. Studies have found discrepancies between plain films and CT imaging in complex anatomy, due to the superior resolution provided by CT [7, 17]. Lateral neck X-rays can be used to assess for adenoid hypertrophy as well but are felt to be inferior to direct visualization with endoscopy. For these reasons, they are not the preferred imaging modality, when imaging is required. Ultrasound has no role in assessing for adenoid hypertrophy or PCRS.

Management

Medical management is the first-line treatment for PCRS. Studies have shown that a topical nasal steroid spray and daily topical nasal saline irrigations are beneficial [2]. Daily saline irrigations have been shown to improve quality of life and Lund-Mackay scores after just six weeks [7]. Additionally, a key component of treatment for PCRS is proper "sinus hygiene." Children should be encouraged to blow their nose and wash their hands regularly [1].

Antibiotics are a standard component of treatment for PCRS. However, the ideal duration of treatment is not well established. Most professional organizations recommend between 10 and 20 days of oral antibiotics [2]. The primary pathogens in PCRS are *Streptococcus pneumoniae, Haemophilus influenzae, Moraxella catarrhalis, and beta-hemolytic Streptococcus pyogenes*. Empiric antibiotic coverage for these pathogens is considered first-line treatment. High-dose amoxicillin, or clindamycin for those with penicillin allergy, is the typical recommendation. Culture-directed antibiotic therapy should be considered when empiric antibiotic treatment fails.

Other therapies such as oral steroids, oral antihistamines, antileukotrienes, antireflux medications, nasal antihistamines, nasal steroid irrigations, nebulized antibiotics, and nebulized steroids have been used in the treatment of PCRS [22, 23].

Surgical intervention is reserved for patients with PCRS who have failed maximal medical therapy. There are several options for surgery in these patients including adenoidectomy and endoscopic sinus surgery (ESS). Given the role that the adenoids play in the pathogenesis of PCRS for children 12 years and younger, adenoidectomy should be considered as a first-line surgical option [2]. It is a simple, well-tolerated procedure. A meta-analysis evaluating the efficacy of adenoidectomy alone in the PCRS population demonstrated a success rate of approximately 70%, in which patients (mean age 5.8 years) had improved sinusitis symptoms after intervention [24]. Although the tonsils are a part of Waldeyer's ring and have similar bacteriology, tonsillectomy is considered an ineffective treatment for PCRS. Adjunctive procedures can also be performed at the same time as the adenoidectomy including ESS and/or balloon sinuplasty [25–27]. Studies have demonstrated that these adjuvant treatments may improve outcomes in the appropriately selected patients [4, 28]. In patients with persistent PCRS despite adenoidectomy, ESS has been shown to be safe and effective [1, 29].

Case Presentation

A 5-year-old male presented with the chief complaint of nasal congestion and recurrent sinusitis. His past medical history included chronic dacryocystitis status post lacrimal probing and stent placement. Symptoms of congestion began 1 year prior to presentation, and over the last six months he developed purulent rhinorrhea and postnasal drip. Antibiotic treatment provided temporary resolution of the rhinorrhea, but the symptoms returned within two to three weeks. In addition to the sinonasal symptoms, he suffers from snoring, restless sleep, and frequent awakenings. Cough is present during times of purulent rhinorrhea and has kept him awake at night but resolves with antibiotic treatment. Skin testing for allergy was negative. He was started on nasal steroid and sinus rinse which were neither well tolerated nor effective.

Physical exam demonstrated a well-appearing child with no notable craniofacial abnormalities. Anterior rhinoscopy revealed midline septum, mucoid discharge, and turbinates without significant hypertrophy. Inspection of the oropharynx revealed 2+ tonsils bilaterally without erythema or exudate. The remainder of the physical exam was unremarkable. Flexible laryngoscopy findings included (Fig. 3.1) patent and well-formed bilateral choanae, midline septum, and a very large adenoid pad. Imaging was not obtained. In this patient, imaging is not necessary to formulate a treatment plan.

The patient was diagnosed with pediatric chronic rhinosinusitis and adenoid hypertrophy refractory to medical management. Adenoidectomy was recommended and performed without complication. At follow-up, the patient had resolution of all sinonasal symptoms as well as sleep disturbance and cough.

Fig. 3.1 Laryngoscopy findings

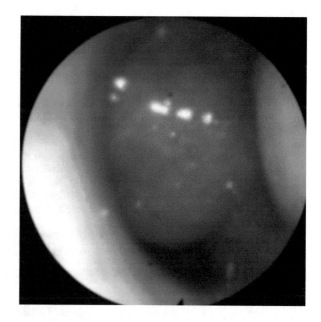

Conclusion

The adenoid pad plays a key role in the etiology of PCRS through several mechanisms. In patients with PCRS who have failed medical management, adenoidectomy should be considered a first-line surgical intervention.

References

1. Heath J, Hartzell L, Putt C, Kennedy JL. Chronic Rhinosinusitis in children: pathophysiology, evaluation, and medical management. Curr Allergy Asthma Rep. 2018;18:37.
2. Brietzke SE, Shin JJ, Choi S, Lee JT, Parikh SR, Pena M, Prager JD, Ramadan H, Veling M, Corrigan M, Rosenfeld RM. Clinical consensus statement: pediatric chronic rhinosinusitis. Otolaryngol Head Neck Surg. 2014;151:542–53.
3. Gilani S, Shin JJ. The burden and visit prevalence of pediatric chronic Rhinosinusitis. Otolaryngol Head Neck Surg. 2017;157:1048–52.
4. Gerber ME, Kennedy AA. Adenoidectomy with balloon catheter Sinuplasty: a randomized trial for pediatric Rhinosinusitis. Laryngoscope. 2018;128:2893–7.
5. Maurizi M, Ottaviani F, Paludetti G, Almadori G, Zappone C. Adenoid hypertrophy and nasal mucociliary clearance in children. A morphological and functional study. Int J Pediatr Otorhinolaryngol. 1984;8:31–41.
6. Arnaoutakis D, Collins WO. Correlation of mucociliary clearance and symptomatology before and after adenoidectomy in children. Int J Pediatr Otorhinolaryngol. 2011;75:1318–21.
7. Belcher R, Virgin F. The role of the adenoids in pediatric chronic Rhinosinusitis. Med Sci (Basel). 2019;7.

8. Cepero R, Smith RJ, Catlin FI, Bressler KL, Furuta GT, Shandera KC. Cystic fibrosis--an otolaryngologic perspective. Otolaryngol Head Neck Surg. 1987;97:356–60.
9. Kerrebijn JD, Poublon RM, Overbeek SE. Nasal and paranasal disease in adult cystic fibrosis patients. Eur Respir J. 1992;5:1239–42.
10. Oomen KP, April MM. Sinonasal manifestations in cystic fibrosis. Int J Otolaryngol. 2012;2012:789572.
11. Wentzel JL, Virella-Lowell I, Schlosser RJ, Soler ZM. Quantitative sinonasal symptom assessment in an unselected pediatric population with cystic fibrosis. Am J Rhinol Allergy. 2015;29:357–61.
12. Sommer JU, Schafer K, Omran H, Olbrich H, Wallmeier J, Blum A, Hormann K, Stuck BA. ENT manifestations in patients with primary ciliary dyskinesia: prevalence and significance of otorhinolaryngologic co-morbidities. Eur Arch Otorhinolaryngol. 2011;268:383–8.
13. Coren ME, Meeks M, Morrison I, Buchdahl RM, Bush A. Primary ciliary dyskinesia: age at diagnosis and symptom history. Acta Paediatr. 2002;91:667–9.
14. Ramadan HH. Chronic rhinosinusitis and bacterial biofilms. Curr Opin Otolaryngol Head Neck Surg. 2006;14:183–6.
15. Eun YG, Park DC, Kim SG, Kim MG, Yeo SG. Immunoglobulins and transcription factors in adenoids of children with otitis media with effusion and chronic rhinosinusitis. Int J Pediatr Otorhinolaryngol. 2009;73:1412–6.
16. Drago L, Pignataro L, Torretta S. Microbiological aspects of acute and chronic pediatric Rhinosinusitis. J Clin Med. 2019;8.
17. Hamilos DL. Pediatric chronic rhinosinusitis. Am J Rhinol Allergy. 2015;29:414–20.
18. Setzen G, Ferguson BJ, Han JK, Rhee JS, Cornelius RS, Froum SJ, Gillman GS, Houser SM, Krakovitz PR, Monfared A, Palmer JN, Rosbe KW, Setzen M, Patel MM. Clinical consensus statement: appropriate use of computed tomography for paranasal sinus disease. Otolaryngol Head Neck Surg. 2012;147:808–16.
19. Peters AT, Spector S, Hsu J, Hamilos DL, Baroody FM, Chandra RK, Grammer LC, Kennedy DW, Cohen NA, Kaliner MA, Wald ER, Karagianis A, Slavin RG. Diagnosis and management of rhinosinusitis: a practice parameter update. Ann Allergy Asthma Immunol. 2014;113:347–85.
20. Mafee MF, Tran BH, Chapa AR. Imaging of rhinosinusitis and its complications: plain film, CT, and MRI. Clin Rev Allergy Immunol. 2006;30:165–86.
21. Muniraj S. Adenoid hypertrophy on MRI. https://radiopaedia.org/cases/adenoid-hypertrophy-on-mri?lang=us.
22. Pai VK, SSS PPD, Mahesh SG. Adenoidectomy versus mometasone furoate nasal spray in treatment of nasal obstruction in children due to adenoid hypertrophy: a comparative study. Inter J Otorhinolaryngol Head Neck Surg. 2019;5(2).
23. Beswick DM, Messner AH, Hwang PH. Pediatric chronic Rhinosinusitis Management in Rhinologists and Pediatric Otolaryngologists. Ann Otol Rhinol Laryngol. 2017;126:634–9.
24. Brietzke SE, Brigger MT. Adenoidectomy outcomes in pediatric rhinosinusitis: a meta-analysis. Int J Pediatr Otorhinolaryngol. 2008;72:1541–5.
25. Ramadan HH. Safety and feasibility of balloon sinuplasty for treatment of chronic rhinosinusitis in children. Ann Otol Rhinol Laryngol. 2009;118:161–5.
26. Ramadan HH, Terrell AM. Balloon catheter sinuplasty and adenoidectomy in children with chronic rhinosinusitis. Ann Otol Rhinol Laryngol. 2010;119:578–82.
27. Ramadan HH, McLaughlin K, Josephson G, Rimell F, Bent J, Parikh SR. Balloon catheter sinuplasty in young children. Allergy Rhinol (Providence). 2010;1:11.
28. Ramadan HH, Cost JL. Outcome of adenoidectomy versus adenoidectomy with maxillary sinus wash for chronic rhinosinusitis in children. Laryngoscope. 2008;118:871–3.
29. Zalzal HG, Makary CA, Ramadan HH. Long-term effectiveness of balloon catheter Sinuplasty in pediatric chronic maxillary sinusitis. Ear Nose Throat J. 2019;98:207–11.

Chapter 4
Asthma and Chronic Rhinosinusitis: Origins and Pathogenesis

Kevin Hur and Kevin C. Welch

> **Key Concepts**
> - Nearly 80% of patients with asthma report some form of rhinitis, and between 22% and 45% are believed to have chronic rhinosinusitis. Conversely, 10–40% of rhinitis patients report coexistent asthma.
> - The prevalence of rhinitis triples the risk for the development of asthma in both atopic and non-atopic patients.
> - Similar pathophysiology results in a unified inflammatory response throughout the upper and lower airway.

Asthma is a chronic inflammatory lower airway condition characterized by reversible airflow obstruction and bronchial hyperreactivity. One of the most commonly diagnosed lower airway diseases, asthma is defined by respiratory symptoms such as wheezing, shortness of breath, chest tightness, and coughing, which vary over time and in severity in conjunction with variable expiratory airflow limitation. There is an association between upper airway diseases such as allergic rhinitis (AR) and chronic rhinosinusitis (CRS) and lower airway diseases such as asthma [1, 2]. Patients with upper airway disease have a higher prevalence of lower airway disease and vice versa. This interrelationship between inflammatory disease of the upper and lower airway has led to the concept that the respiratory system functions as an integrated unit termed "the unified airway." [2–4] In this model, diseases which cause inflammation in one part of the airway will likely stimulate a similar reaction throughout the rest of the airway. In this chapter, we will review the relationship between asthma and CRS.

K. Hur · K. C. Welch (✉)
Department of Otolaryngology - Head and Neck Surgery, Feinberg School of Medicine, Northwestern University, Chicago, IL, USA
e-mail: kwelch2@nm.org

© Springer Nature Switzerland AG 2020
D. A. Gudis, R. J. Schlosser (eds.), *The Unified Airway*,
https://doi.org/10.1007/978-3-030-50330-7_4

Epidemiology

With an annual economic burden of $56 billion in the United States, the prevalence of asthma has increased over the last few decades with a higher prevalence in developed countries [5]. The global prevalence of doctor-diagnosed asthma is 4.3%, while in the United States, epidemiologic studies by the Centers for Disease Control and Prevention have reported a prevalence of 8.4% in children and 8.1% in adults [6]. Asthma is the most common noncommunicable disease in children, and there are health disparities in asthma morbidity and mortality with respect to race, ethnicity, and income [7]. Women have a higher prevalence and greater severity of asthma in adulthood compared to men [8]. African American children have higher rates of asthma, hospitalizations for asthma, and asthma-related mortality compared to white children, which may stem from several factors such as healthcare access, health literacy, clinical bias, and genetic risk factors [9].

Epidemiologic evidence also supports the coexistence of asthma and other upper airway conditions, as previously mentioned. For instance, nearly 80% of patients with asthma report some form of rhinitis, defined as irritation and inflammation of the mucous membranes of the nose. Conversely, 10–40% of rhinitis patients report coexistent asthma [10]. The presence of rhinitis triples the risk for the development of asthma in both atopic and non-atopic individuals [11]. In a study by Linneberg et al., individuals with allergic rhinitis who were sensitized to perennial allergens were found to have a significantly higher likelihood of developing asthma than individuals who were sensitized to seasonal allergens [12].

In the general population, the prevalence of CRS is estimated to affect up to 12% of adults [13, 14]. However, among asthmatics, the prevalence of CRS is estimated to be between 22% and 45% [15–17]. CRS is associated with more severe asthma, especially in patients with chronic rhinosinusitis with nasal polyposis (CRSwNP) [18]. Among patients with CRS, asthmatic patients are more likely to have nasal polyps [19]. The presence of nasal polyps is similarly associated with more severe sinus symptoms, including facial pain and pressure and hyposmia, relative to CRS without polyps (CRSsNP) [20]. In a recent cluster analysis performed by the Severe Asthma Research Program, nearly half of the patients with the most severe burden of disease had a history of previous endoscopic sinus surgery (ESS), suggesting that CRS refractory to medical management is associated with more severe forms of asthma [17].

Pathophysiology

The etiology of asthma is not currently known, but several risk factors have been identified along the spectrum from genetics to environmental factors that are associated with asthma development. Genetics has long been recognized as a risk factor, with the observation that the offspring of asthmatic parents are at increased risk of developing asthma [21, 22]. Hundreds of genetic variants have already been identified through genome sequencing that are associated with an increased risk of asthma

[23]. Epigenetic variations, or modifications of gene expression without alterations in the underlying nucleotide sequence, can also lead to the dysregulation of inflammation seen in asthma [24]. Respiratory infections, environmental exposures such as tobacco smoke, and atopic conditions all have been strongly associated with an increased risk of developing asthma as well. Other factors theorized to play a role include stress, dietary changes, chemical exposure, vitamin D level abnormalities, and the microbiome [25–29]. The interaction of these multiple environmental risk factors with the broad diversity of genetic and epigenetic variants associated with asthma eventually leads to the pathophysiologic changes which result in the classic clinical symptoms of asthma [30].

In patients with asthma, allergens, pollutants, irritants, and microbes elicit various inflammatory cascades in the lower airway that are mediated by multiple cell types including dendritic cells, mast cells, eosinophils, T lymphocytes, macrophages, neutrophils, and epithelial cells [6]. Multiple pathological changes occur in the lower airway epithelium and submucosa referred to as airway remodeling. Epithelial changes include goblet cell hyperplasia and increases in epithelial mucin stores. Changes in the submucosa include subepithelial fibrosis with collagen deposition, increased volume of submucosal glands, hypertrophy and hyperplasia of smooth muscle cells, and angiogenesis [31]. These changes are initially reversible with treatment, but with continued inflammation, irreversible remodeling of the lower airway can occur. The cellular alterations predispose individuals to exacerbations by decreasing the airway lumen caliber and increasing sensitivity toward inhaled irritants, which is commonly labeled as "airway hyperresponsiveness." Similar histopathological changes are often observed in CRS, including sinonasal mucosal thickening, submucosal gland hypertrophy, collagen deposition, and basement membrane thickening [32].

Despite the common histopathological changes seen in asthmatic patients, asthma severity varies greatly between patients. This phenotypic heterogeneity has been analyzed with cluster analysis and found to vary based on age, gender, atopy, lung function, healthcare utilization, and body mass index [17, 33]. However, phenotypic heterogeneity is limited in informing our understanding of pathophysiological mechanisms as the clinical severity of asthma can be a result of several distinct mechanistic pathways, termed endotypes [31]. Therefore, there is growing research into elucidating the various asthma endotypes, which may spur the development of more personalized treatment for this heterogeneous disease.

Currently, asthma can be categorized into two general endotypes: those with increased levels of type 2 inflammation (Th2-high) and those without high levels of type 2 inflammation (Th2-low). Type 2 inflammation is a distinct immune response regulated by a type of CD4 T cell called a T helper 2 cell lymphocyte (Th2). Th2 cells are characterized by a specific cytokine profile, mainly IL-4, IL-5, and IL-13. Type 2 inflammation is commonly identified in allergic disease, eosinophilic disorders, and parasitic infections. Patients with Th2-high asthma have eosinophilia and an increased number of airway mast cells which is driven by dendritic cell stimulation of Th2 cells [34]. The downstream effects of a Th2 response are the release of histamine and leukotrienes causing bronchoconstriction. This inflammatory pathway is perpetuated and maintained by IL-25, IL-33, and thymic stromal lymphopoietin which are produced by dendritic and epithelial cells [35].

The clinical relevance of distinguishing between Th2-high asthma and Th2-low asthma is the response to treatment with inhaled corticosteroids. Th2-high asthma generally is responsive to corticosteroids, while Th2-low asthma is not [36]. Nevertheless, there are subgroups of patients with Th2-high asthma who have persistent symptoms that cannot be controlled with corticosteroids that may be secondary to very high levels of type 2 inflammation or innate steroid resistance [31]. Our understanding of asthma endotypes is still developing, and there are likely several endotypes that have yet to be defined or discovered.

The pathophysiology of CRS is similar to that seen in asthma. About 85% of Western CRSwNP exhibits type 2 inflammation, which explains the effectiveness of corticosteroids for CRSwNP and the potential benefit of biologics which target elements of this pathway [37, 38]. The process begins with epithelial signals that stimulate type 2 innate lymphocytes (ILC2 cells) and Th2 differentiation with the production of cytokines IL-4, IL-5, and IL-13. These cytokines invoke a cascade leading to the infiltration and/or activation of large numbers of eosinophils, mast cells, and basophils. In Asian countries, patients with CRSwNP tend to have a more neutrophilic cellular predominance. Less type 2 inflammation is observed in Asian CRSwNP, which exhibit predominantly type 1 and type 3 inflammation. In parallel, ILC1 and ILC3 cells are activated as well as the corresponding Th1 and Th17 subsets with release of the canonical cytokines IFN-γ and IL-17, respectively [39]. Type 2 cytokines IL-4, IL-5, and IL-13 influence several biological processes including immunoglobulin class switching to IgE, IgG4 mucous production, inflammatory cell chemotaxis with upregulation of vascular cell adhesion molecule-1 (VCAM-1), and the activation of eosinophils [40]. The ILC cells in general function as the first-line defenders in the airway epithelial barrier. The epithelial signals to ILC2s are well characterized, and these cells are also important sources of type 2 cytokines in CRSwNP, in addition to the Th2 lymphocytes [41–43].

Clinical Presentation

The four cardinal symptoms of asthma include wheezing, shortness of breath, chest tightness, and coughing. Clinicians should inquire about these symptoms if there is suspicion for asthma. However, the underlying inflammation of asthma may be present in the absence of symptoms, and symptoms may also vary in intensity and frequency in an individual over time, making the diagnosis difficult [44]. Wheezing is a more specific symptom than cough but is less common and may indicate worsening of bronchospasm. Chest tightness and shortness of breath generally occur in more severe asthma. In a sample of 1257 New Zealanders, researchers found that wheezing and dyspnea were the single best predictor of diagnosed asthma with a sensitivity of 82% and a specificity of 90% [45].

In addition to screening for the cardinal symptoms of asthma, healthcare providers should also assess for any triggers or antecedent events that elicit these symptoms. These triggers can include nonallergic causes such as viral infections, smoking, chemical irritants, or medications, as well as allergic or atopic diseases

[46]. The timing of symptoms in a patient's life may also be insightful for the provider. Allergic disease diminishes with age and therefore is less likely an inflammatory trigger in older adults [44].

The physical exam should include a head and neck exam with nasal endoscopy and laryngoscopy as well as a careful respiratory exam that includes auscultation. Physical exam findings suggestive of asthma include a dry cough and end-expiratory wheezes on chest auscultation. In patients with an acute exacerbation, patients often will display accessory muscle use, tachypnea, and in severe cases cyanosis [46]. However, providers should remember that the physical exam can be normal even in those with severe disease due to the variability in symptom expression. Therefore, a negative physical exam cannot exclude an asthma diagnosis.

Due to the variability in the clinical presentation, objective testing plays a major role in the diagnosis of asthma. There are two components necessary for an objective diagnosis: (1) evidence of airway obstruction and (2) demonstration of reversibility in degree of obstruction [47]. The primary procedure for determining these components is through pulmonary function testing, with spirometry being the method of choice. In spirometry testing, the patient takes a full inhalation and rapidly exhales into a measurement device. Airflow measurements include the forced expiratory volume in 1 second (FEV1) and the forced vital capacity (FVC) [46]. A reduction of the FEV1/FVC ratio is generally considered obstruction if it is below 0.75 in adults or 0.9 in children, though a comparison to normative values based on the demographics of the patient should be performed [47]. A value less than 80% of the predicted value is considered diagnostic of asthma. Variability in lung function can be determined by a change in the FEV1 greater than 12% after a bronchodilator reversibility test or a four-week trial of anti-inflammatory controller therapy [46].

In an asthmatic patient with subclinical or intermittent disease, pulmonary function testing may be nondiagnostic, and therefore other supportive testing methods should be considered such as bronchial provocation. Nonpharmacological bronchial provocation methods include exercising or eucapnic voluntary ventilation. A decrease in FEV1 by at least 10% may be considered a positive result. Pharmacologic bronchial challenge testing involves the administration of increasing doses of methacholine or histamine, with a 20% change in FEV1 considered a positive result [47]. Other methods of testing include exhaled nitric oxide testing, which uses the presence of nitric oxide as a proxy for airway inflammation. Skin testing or in vitro serum IgE tests may be useful in diagnosing atopic asthma or possible triggers for the patient.

Chronic rhinosinusitis (CRS) is classically defined as inflammation of the nose and paranasal sinuses for at least 12 weeks in duration and affects about 3.0–16.1% of the Western population based on sinus radiology and symptomatology [13, 14, 48, 49]. Diagnosis of CRS according to the EPOS 2012 guidelines includes the presence of two or more of the following symptoms for at least 12 weeks in duration: (1) nasal blockage/obstruction/congestion, (2) nasal discharge, (3) facial pain/pressure, and (4) reduction or loss of smell. In addition, objective confirmation of inflammation by radiography (e.g., abnormal sinus CT) or nasal endoscopy (e.g., mucopurulent discharge, mucosal edema, or polyps) is necessary [49].

CRS encompasses a heterogeneous group of conditions with differing pathophysiologies. Traditionally, two main subgroups have been described: CRS with polyps (CRSwNP) and CRS without nasal polyps (CRSsNP). The differentiation between the two groups is made by the identification of nasal polyps on nasal endoscopy. However, within these main categories of CRS are subgroups of specific clinical phenotypes that are associated with infectious, genetic, metabolic, or immunologic diseases. Examples of CRS phenotypes with distinct clinical features include aspirin-exacerbated respiratory disease (AERD), allergic fungal rhinosinusitis, cystic fibrosis, odontogenic rhinosinusitis, immunodeficiency, primary ciliary dyskinesias, and eosinophilic granulomatosis with polyangiitis.

The coexistence of both asthma and CRS in the same patient appears to influence the severity of both the upper and lower airway diseases [50]. Asthma can develop either in childhood or as an adult, but CRS is more strongly linked with adult-onset asthma [51]. Patients with adult-onset asthma are also more likely to develop CRSwNP, require more treatment for CRS, and have poorer physical function than those with childhood-onset asthma [52]. Among CRS patients seen at a tertiary center, those with comorbid asthma had significantly worse sinus CT and nasal endoscopic scores compared to patients with CRS without asthma [53, 54]. A correlation between the severity of asthma and severity of CRS has been reported in a study of 187 CRS patients at an academic center [55]. In a cluster analysis of 726 asthma subjects, phenotypes that were classified as severe asthma based on severe airflow limitations at baseline had the highest percentage of reported sinus disease [17]. Advanced sinus disease has been identified as a strong independent risk factor for having more severe asthma [56, 57]. Patients with both CRS and asthma have worse lung function on spirometry and quality of life compared to patients with asthma alone [16]. Severe CRS is also an independent risk factor for frequent asthma exacerbations [56]. CRS and asthma appear to significantly influence the severity each other, and therefore the screening and accurate diagnosis of both entities in patients is crucial for the practicing physician.

Aspirin-Exacerbated Respiratory Disease

Aspirin-exacerbated respiratory disease (AERD) is a disease that affects both the upper and lower airways and is characterized by the clinical triad of nasal polyps, asthma, and sensitivity to cyclooxygenase type 1 inhibitors. The upper and lower airways are exacerbated by aspirin or other nonsteroidal anti-inflammatory drug (NSAID) ingestion that inhibits cyclooxygenase type 1 [58]. Although the pathophysiology of AERD is still being elucidated, this unique clinical syndrome involves the dysregulation of arachidonic acid metabolism (higher production of cysteinyl leukotrienes and prostaglandin D2 with lower levels of prostaglandin E2) and increased activation of type 2 effector immune cells, such as eosinophils and mast cells, in addition to genetic and epigenetic factors. Other cells such as epithelial cells, ILC2s, basophils, and platelets are also believed to be activated and involved in the pathogenesis of AERD [59, 60].

The prevalence of AERD is between 7% and 21% among adult asthma patients and between 9 and 16% of CRSwNP patients [61, 62]. A 2015 systematic review of 1770 publications concluded that the prevalence of AERD was 7% in those with asthma, 15% in those with severe asthma, and 10% in those with CRSwNP. Interestingly, the prevalence of AERD is mostly based on studies of Western and European populations [63]. In Asian populations, the prevalence of AERD has been found to be much lower for unclear reasons [64].

The clinical diagnosis of AERD relies on the confirmation of the three major components of the disease: CRSwNP, asthma, and hypersensitivity to aspirin/NSAIDs. These components can be identified with a detailed clinical history and examination that should include endoscopy, radiologic imaging, spirometry, and an aspirin challenge.

Patients with AERD tend to present with a more severe clinical presentation compared to other phenotypes of CRS. Typical nasal symptoms of CRS including rhinorrhea and nasal congestion are usually the first symptoms to manifest in the course of the disease and may be difficult to distinguish from other CRS phenotypes. However, the degree of sinonasal inflammation found on diagnostic CT scans has been reported to be significantly higher in severity for AERD patients compared to CRSwNP with asthma or CRSsNP patients. AERD patients undergo a significantly higher number of sinus surgeries compared to other CRSwNP patients, thus implying that AERD patients are more likely to have disease recurrence [61].

Asthma symptoms may develop before or after the presentation of upper airway disease. AERD patients have significantly decreased FEV1 compared to nonaspirin-sensitive CRS patients with asthma [61, 65]. The unified airway hypothesis suggests that upper and lower airway diseases are linked, and an increase in disease severity of the upper airway will likely impact the severity of disease in the lower airway. Therefore, it is reasonable to conclude that since AERD patients are more likely to have more severe and refractory sinonasal disease, they also are more likely to have more severe lower airway disease.

The key defining feature of AERD that distinguishes it from other CRS phenotypes is aspirin/NSAID hypersensitivity, which may develop gradually and be difficult to diagnose. A typical presentation of hypersensitivity includes symptoms of rhinorrhea, epiphora, conjunctival edema, nasal congestion, laryngospasm, or bronchospasm, typically occurring within hours after ingestion of aspirin/NSAIDs. A history of an asthma attack following ingestion of aspirin or other NSAIDs is also suggestive of a diagnosis. However, a clinical history is not necessarily definitive in the diagnosis of an aspirin/NSAID hypersensitivity. In one study, 16% of patients who reported a history of an asthma attack after ingesting aspirin/NSAIDs had a negative oral aspirin provocation challenge. Furthermore, the same study reported that in patients who presented with nasal polyps, CRS, asthma, and a history of avoiding aspirin/NSAIDs, only 43% had a positive oral aspirin challenge [66]. Therefore, an aspirin challenge remains the gold standard for diagnosing AERD as there is no other available form of laboratory testing with similar precision and accuracy available to diagnose hypersensitivity. Several methods of provocation challenges have been described, including oral, bronchial inhalation, nasal inhalation, and intravenous [58].

Medical Management and Outcomes

Asthma is a chronic disease with no known cure. The goal of contemporary asthma management is to establish control of the disease, improve symptoms, and improve quality of life. Therapeutic options to eliminate and reverse the underlying inflammatory pathophysiologic changes are lacking at this time.

The goal of asthma management is to maintain control over symptoms over time with the minimal amount of medication [46]. Symptom control includes maintaining normal activities such as exercise, preventing asthma exacerbations, avoiding adverse effects from asthma medications, and preventing asthma mortality [67]. To achieve this goal, a stepwise approach is performed in which pharmacological treatment is continually adjusted based on serial assessments of response to therapy [6].

Medications for asthma are broadly categorized into two groups: control medications, used to achieve and maintain baseline control of persistent asthma, and rescue medications used to treat acute symptoms and exacerbations. The initial pharmacological regimen is selected based on disease severity, which is classified as intermittent, mild persistent, moderate persistent, and severe persistent. Severity class is determined by a combination of frequency of symptoms and lung function results. For intermittent asthma, a short-acting beta-2 agonist (SABA), which is a rescue medication, can be utilized as symptoms arise and can generally control these infrequent episodes. For mild persistent asthma, low-dose inhaled corticosteroids (ICS) are the foundation of treatment. ICS have been shown to reduce asthma symptoms, increase lung function, improve quality of life, and reduce the risks of exacerbations, asthma-related hospitalizations, and asthma-related death [68, 69]. With increasing severity, higher doses of ICS are used along with long-acting beta-2 agonist (LABA) combination medications. Lastly, patients with persistent symptoms or exacerbations despite optimized therapeutic regimens can be considered for systemic therapy such as oral corticosteroids and biologics. Several biologics have recently been introduced in the treatment of asthma including omalizumab, mepolizumab, reslizumab, benralizumab, and dupilumab [70]. Anti-IgE (omalizumab) therapy has shown benefit for those with severe allergic asthma [71]. Anti-IL-5 (mepolizumab, reslizumab), anti-IL-5 receptor (benralizumab), and anti-IL-4 receptor (dupilumab) therapy can be used for treatment of uncontrolled, severe eosinophilic asthma [72, 73].

The medical management of CRS generally includes a combination of nasal saline irrigations, topical steroids, antibiotics, and/or oral corticosteroids depending on the presence of polyps [49]. Sinus surgery is generally considered for CRS patients who have failed appropriate medical therapy. The use of corticosteroids for the management of CRS is supported by a high level of evidence, with particularly strong evidence for cases of CRSwNP [74–76]. Whether the medical treatment of either disease impacts the course of the other is unclear. A double-blind placebo-controlled trial of nasal mometasone spray in adults and children with uncontrolled asthma found that there was no improvement in asthma control [77]. The study concluded that treatment of sinonasal disease in asthmatic patients should be guided by sinonasal symptoms and severity of sinus disease rather than for asthma control.

The effects of montelukast, a leukotriene receptor antagonist, on patients with nasal polyposis and asthma are also unclear. In a placebo-controlled trial of 24 patients with nasal polyps and controlled asthma, those who received daily montelukast for 6 weeks had significant improvements in nasal symptom score and airflow limitation as well as a reduction in inflammatory mediators in nasal lavage samples [78]. However, a separate trial of montelukast as an add-on therapy to topical and inhaled corticosteroids in patients with asthma and nasal polyps reported that while there was subjective improvement in nasal polyposis and asthma symptoms, there was no objective improvement in acoustic rhinometry, nasal inspiratory peak flow, or nitric oxide levels compared to pre-montelukast therapy [79].

Recent immunomodulatory biologics have been demonstrated to improve both asthma and eosinophilic CRS. At the time of publishing, dupilumab has been approved for the treatment of both asthma and CRSwNP following phase II and phase III trials, and several other biologics are also being investigated [80, 81]. The medication is self-injected biweekly by the patient either in the thigh or abdomen. Dupilumab was initially approved in 2017 for the treatment of moderate-to-severe atopic dermatitis and in 2018 for the treatment of moderate-to-severe refractory eosinophilic or steroid-dependent asthma [82, 83]. The biologic is a human IgG4 monoclonal antibody directed against the IL-4 receptor-α (IL4Rα) subunit. Binding of dupilumab to the IL-4Ra subunit inhibits the signaling of both IL-4 and IL-13, two cytokines in the type 2 inflammatory pathway key to the pathophysiology of atopic dermatitis, asthma, and CRSwNP.

Surgical Management and Outcomes

The impact that the surgical management of the upper airway has on the lower airway has been discussed in the literature for at least a century. In the 1920s, the majority of patients in a series of 13 asthmatic individuals who underwent ESS had worsening of their lower respiratory tract symptoms, which led to the initial theory that asthma was adversely affected by ESS [84]. However, in the 1970s, further studies demonstrated that polypectomy in patients with asthma did not appear to alter subjective asthma symptoms [85, 86]. Then in 1999, a qualitative review of the literature suggested that ESS appeared to improve asthma severity in two-thirds of patients by reducing the use of medications and hospitalizations while improving pulmonary function tests [84]. While that study did not systematically review the available literature, future studies continued to support the theory that surgical management of CRS improves asthma control with validated asthma outcome measures.

A quantitative meta-analysis of asthma outcomes in patients with CRS following ESS was published in 2013 which reported that ESS improved almost all clinical asthma outcome measures: improved overall asthma control in 76.1% of patients, decreased frequency of asthma attacks in 84.8% of patients, decreased number of hospitalizations in 64.4%, decreased use of oral corticosteroids in 72.8%, decreased inhaled corticosteroid use in 28.5%, and decreased bronchodilator use in 36.3% of patients [87]. However, there was no improvement in pulmonary function testing [87]. A study in Taiwan of 28 patients with asthma and CRS who underwent ESS found that patients with severe asthma, defined as requiring continuous or near-continuous use of oral corticosteroids, had significantly improved asthma control test (ACT) scores and lung function testing compared to patients with non-severe asthma [88]. Similarly, a multi-institutional prospective study of patients with CRS and comorbid asthma who underwent ESS showed improved scores on the Mini-Asthma Quality of Life Questionnaire and the ACT with approximately half of patients with uncontrolled asthma improving after surgery [89]. However, a prospective Chinese study of 27 CRS patients with asthma who underwent ESS reported no reduction in the use of asthma medication up to 3 years postoperatively and no improvement in pulmonary function testing [90]. It should be noted that only 11% of patients in the study cohort had poorly controlled asthma. Based on these recent studies, the benefit of ESS in patients with CRS and asthma seems to be most significant in patients with poorly controlled asthma in the preoperative setting.

The timing of surgery may also play a role in CRS patients with asthma. CRS patients who experience delayed sinus surgery demonstrate less improvement in Sinonasal Outcome Test 22-Item Questionnaire (SNOT-22) scores than those who receive prompt surgical intervention, and asthma has been identified as a risk factor for delayed surgical intervention [91]. A retrospective analysis of a claims database of CRS patients who underwent ESS in the United States in 2010 found that patients with ongoing, medically recalcitrant CRS had a 5% increased risk annually of developing asthma, which only declined after surgery [92]. Therefore, surgical management of CRS may significantly impact the development and the control of asthma, especially severe uncontrolled asthma.

Impact of Rhinologic Interventions on Medical Disorder

Medical and surgical rhinologic interventions to treat CRS have been increasingly reported to improve asthma control [6]. In a study from Japan, CRS patients with asthma who underwent ESS had improvement in their asthma symptoms, peak flow, and medication score [93]. However, in a recent systematic review evaluating various medical and surgical interventions for CRSwNP and comorbid asthma, the efficacy of ESS and systemic anti-inflammatory drugs did not lead to significant improvement in asthma outcomes. This study did note that a major limitation of the review was the lack of high-quality trials [94]. The conflicting results of studies evaluating the impact of rhinologic interventions on asthma are likely due to the heterogeneous nature of both diseases. These studies likely have cohorts that contain a spectrum of both CRS and asthma endotypes that respond differently to the currently available therapeutic options. There are likely certain asthma subtypes that will improve with rhinologic interventions and certain subtypes that will not. Future studies are necessary to clarify which patients will benefit.

Case Presentation

To illustrate the unified nature of asthma and CRSwNP, the case of a 63-year-old male is reviewed. This patient had a 16-year history of sinonasal complaints consisting of right greater than left nasal obstruction, continuous discolored nasal discharge, anosmia, and midface as well as frontal pressure. He had undergone two previous sinus surgeries and had been treated by three prior otolaryngologists with antibiotics, topical steroid sprays, steroid irrigations, and systemic steroids. Additionally, he reported a history of allergic rhinitis to multiple inhalant allergens, having been tested 10 years prior to his consultation with us. His review of systems was significant for cough, but he did not carry a formal diagnosis of asthma. He denied sensitivity to aspirin or NSAIDs. His physical examination was remarkable for bilateral thick clear nasal drainage, pale turbinates, and polyps. Nasal endoscopy demonstrated grade 3/4 polyps on both sides as well as significant middle meatus edema. A CT scan was obtained in the office, and this demonstrated a Lund-MacKay score of 23/24 with opacification in all sinuses, except the left maxillary sinus (Fig. 4.1). The patient was sent for an allergy/immunology evaluation. His serology was notable for an IgE of 344 (<114.0) and an absolute eosinophil count of 1300

Fig. 4.1 A representative coronal CT scan of the patient's sinuses. The representative scan reveals opacification of the sinuses as well as some residual partitions in the ethmoid cavities. There are no orbital or skull base deformations, but the findings of the CT represent severe recurrent CRSwNP

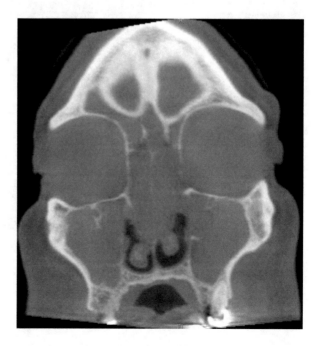

(p/c-ANCA negative). Pulmonary function testing revealed an FVC of 2.77 (55% predicted) and an FEV1 of 2.14 (57% predicted).

Given the prior history of ESS, the recurrence and persistence of diffuse inflammatory mucosal disease, and the need to improve access for topical therapy, the patient elected to undergo revision ESS. In addition to the completion ESS, the patient underwent a modified Lothrop/Draf III and bilateral modified endoscopic medial maxillectomies to improve the delivery of postoperative steroid irrigations and improve access for debridements when necessary. The surgery was uneventful, and the patient was placed on a 4-week tapering dose of prednisone and immediately on mometasone 1 mg BID topical sinus irrigations.

Two years after the surgery, the patient was seen in follow-up. The patient reported good symptom control with occasional mildly symptomatic clear drainage, improved sense of smell, absence of obstruction, and elimination of facial pressure. Endoscopy revealed widely patent sinuses (Fig. 4.2). Moreover, he reported good asthma control without shortness of breath, coughing, or wheezing. His pulmonary function testing, performed nearly 2 years after surgery, revealed vast improvements in his asthma as well with an FVC of 3.58 (72% predicted) and an FEV1 of 2.74 (74% predicted). He has not required any prednisone for asthma exacerbations since the surgery. He is maintained on a fluticasone/salmeterol inhaler for his asthma and 1 mg mometasone irrigations BID.

Fig. 4.2 A postoperative endoscopic view of the frontal sinus taken 2 years after surgery. Endoscopy of this Lothrop/Draf III cavity reveals otherwise normal-appearing mucosa without significant edema, scarring, infection, or recurrent polyposis

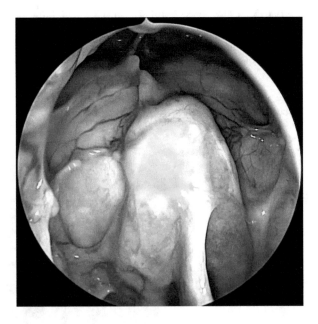

Conclusion

There is a strong relationship between asthma and CRS that can be observed clinically. While both diseases encompass a heterogeneous group of endotypes and phenotypes, the pathophysiologic mechanisms of the underlying inflammatory processes of asthma and CRS share many similarities. Therefore, it is not surprising that there is growing evidence that the medical and surgical management of the upper airway provides clinical benefit to the lower airway as well in the form of improved asthma symptoms and control, especially in patients with severe asthma. The accurate diagnosis and treatment of both upper and lower airway diseases is necessary for the optimal management of CRS and asthma.

References

1. Greenberger PA. Allergic rhinitis and asthma connection: treatment implications. Allergy Asthma Proc. 2008;29:557–64.
2. Slavin RG. The upper and lower airways: the epidemiological and pathophysiological connection. Allergy Asthma Proc. 2008;29:553–6.
3. Krouse JH. The unified airway--conceptual framework. Otolaryngol Clin N Am. 2008;41:257–66.
4. Licari A, Castagnoli R, Denicolo CF, Rossini L, Marseglia A, Marseglia GL. The nose and the lung: united airway disease? Front Pediatr. 2017;5:44.
5. Loftus PA, Wise SK. Epidemiology and economic burden of asthma. Int Forum Allergy Rhinol. 2015;5(Suppl 1):S7–10.
6. Massoth L, Anderson C, McKinney KA. Asthma and chronic Rhinosinusitis: diagnosis and medical management. Med Sci (Basel). 2019;7.
7. Bryant-Stephens T. Asthma disparities in urban environments. J Allergy Clin Immunol. 2009;123:1199–206.. quiz 1207-1198
8. Postma DS. Gender differences in asthma development and progression. Gend Med. 2007;4. Suppl B:S133–46.
9. Hughes HK, Matsui EC, Tschudy MM, Pollack CE, Keet CA. Pediatric asthma health disparities: race, hardship, housing, and asthma in a National Survey. Acad Pediatr. 2017;17:127–34.
10. Bousquet J, Khaltaev N. Cruz AAet al. Allergic rhinitis and its impact on asthma (ARIA) 2008 update (in collaboration with the World Health Organization, GA(2)LEN and AllerGen). Allergy. 2008;63(Suppl 86):8–160.
11. Guerra S, Sherrill DL, Martinez FD, Barbee RA. Rhinitis as an independent risk factor for adult-onset asthma. J Allergy Clin Immunol. 2002;109:419–25.
12. Linneberg A, Henrik Nielsen N. Frolund let al. The link between allergic rhinitis and allergic asthma: a prospective population-based study. The Copenhagen allergy study. Allergy. 2002;57:1048–52.
13. Dietz de Loos D, Lourijsen ES. Wildeman MAMet al. Prevalence of chronic rhinosinusitis in the general population based on sinus radiology and symptomatology. J Allergy Clin Immunol. 2019;143:1207–14.

14. Hirsch AG, Nordberg C, Bandeen-Roche K, et al. Radiologic sinus inflammation and symptoms of chronic rhinosinusitis in a population-based sample. Allergy. 2019; https://doi.org/10.1111/all.14106.

15. Liou A, Grubb JR, Schechtman KB, Hamilos DL. Causative and contributive factors to asthma severity and patterns of medication use in patients seeking specialized asthma care. Chest. 2003;124:1781–8.

16. Ek A, Middelveld RJ. Bertilsson Het al. Chronic rhinosinusitis in asthma is a negative predictor of quality of life: results from the Swedish GA(2)LEN survey. Allergy. 2013;68:1314–21.

17. Moore WC, Meyers DA. Wenzel SEet al. Identification of asthma phenotypes using cluster analysis in the severe asthma research program. Am J Respir Crit Care Med. 2010;181:315–23.

18. Hamilos DL. Chronic Rhinosinusitis in patients with cystic fibrosis. J Allergy Clin Immunol Pract. 2016;4:605–12.

19. Pearlman AN, Chandra RK. Chang Det al. Relationships between severity of chronic rhinosinusitis and nasal polyposis, asthma, and atopy. Am J Rhinol Allergy. 2009;23:145–8.

20. Palmer JN, Messina JC, Biletch R, Grosel K, Mahmoud RA. A cross-sectional, population-based survey of U.S. adults with symptoms of chronic rhinosinusitis. Allergy Asthma Proc. 2019 Jan 14;40(1):48–56.

21. Ober C, Yao TC. The genetics of asthma and allergic disease: a 21st century perspective. Immunol Rev. 2011;242:10–30.

22. Lim RH, Kobzik L, Dahl M. Risk for asthma in offspring of asthmatic mothers versus fathers: a meta-analysis. PLoS One. 2010;5:e10134.

23. Holloway JW, Yang IA, Holgate ST. Genetics of allergic disease. J Allergy Clin Immunol. 2010;125:S81–94.

24. Harb H, Renz H. Update on epigenetics in allergic disease. J Allergy Clin Immunol. 2015;135:15–24.

25. Bunyavanich S, Schadt EE. Systems biology of asthma and allergic diseases: a multiscale approach. J Allergy Clin Immunol. 2015;135:31–42.

26. Raissy H, Blake K. Vitamin D and asthma: association, causality, or intervention? Pediatr Allergy Immunol Pulmonol. 2015;28:60–2.

27. Smit LA, Lenters V. Hoyer BBet al. Prenatal exposure to environmental chemical contaminants and asthma and eczema in school-age children. Allergy. 2015;70:653–60.

28. DeChristopher LR, Uribarri J, Tucker KL. Intakes of apple juice, fruit drinks and soda are associated with prevalent asthma in US children aged 2-9 years. Public Health Nutr. 2016;19:123–30.

29. Wong KO, Hunter Rowe B, Douwes J, Senthilselvan A. Asthma and wheezing are associated with depression and anxiety in adults: an analysis from 54 countries. Pulm Med. 2013;2013:929028.

30. Mims JW. Asthma: definitions and pathophysiology. Int Forum Allergy Rhinol. 2015;5(Suppl 1):S2–6.

31. Fahy JV. Type 2 inflammation in asthma--present in most, absent in many. Nat Rev Immunol. 2015;15:57–65.

32. Ponikau JU, Sherris DA. Kephart GMet al. Features of airway remodeling and eosinophilic inflammation in chronic rhinosinusitis: is the histopathology similar to asthma? J Allergy Clin Immunol. 2003;112:877–82.

33. Haldar P, Pavord ID. Shaw DEet al. Cluster analysis and clinical asthma phenotypes. Am J Respir Crit Care Med. 2008;178:218–24.

34. Dougherty RH, Sidhu SS, Raman K, et al. Accumulation of intraepithelial mast cells with a unique protease phenotype in T(H)2-high asthma. J Allergy Clin Immunol. 2010;125:1046–1053 e1048.

35. Gans MD, Gavrilova T. Understanding the immunology of asthma: Pathophysiology, biomarkers, and treatments for asthma endotypes. Paediatr Respir Rev. 2019;S1526–0542(19)30081–8.

36. Woodruff PG, Modrek B. Choy DFet al. T-helper type 2-driven inflammation defines major subphenotypes of asthma. Am J Respir Crit Care Med. 2009;180:388–95.

37. Stevens WW, Peters AT, Tan BK, et al. Associations Between Inflammatory Endotypes and Clinical Presentations in Chronic Rhinosinusitis. J Allergy Clin Immunol Pract. 2019;7:2812–2820 e2813.
38. Tomassen P, Vandeplas G, Van Zele T, et al. Inflammatory endotypes of chronic rhinosinusitis based on cluster analysis of biomarkers. J Allergy Clin Immunol. 2016;137:1449–1456 e1444.
39. Bachert C, Zhang L, Gevaert P. Current and future treatment options for adult chronic rhinosinusitis: focus on nasal polyposis. J Allergy Clin Immunol. 2015;136:1431–40.
40. Lavigne P, Lee SE. Immunomodulators in chronic rhinosinusitis. World J Otorhinolaryngol Head Neck Surg. 2018;4:186–92.
41. Shaw JL, Fakhri S. Citardi MJet al. IL-33-responsive innate lymphoid cells are an important source of IL-13 in chronic rhinosinusitis with nasal polyps. Am J Respir Crit Care Med. 2013;188:432–9.
42. Mjosberg JM, Trifari S, Crellin NK, et al. Human IL-25- and IL-33-responsive type 2 innate lymphoid cells are defined by expression of CRTH2 and CD161. Nat Immunol. 2011;12:1055–62.
43. Nagarkar DR, Poposki JA, Tan BK, et al. Thymic stromal lymphopoietin activity is increased in nasal polyps of patients with chronic rhinosinusitis. J Allergy Clin Immunol. 2013;132:593–600 e512.
44. Reisacher WR. Asthma and the otolaryngologist. Int Forum Allergy Rhinol. 2014;4(Suppl 2):S70–3.
45. Sistek D, Wickens K, Amstrong R, D'Souza W, Town I, Crane J. Predictive value of respiratory symptoms and bronchial hyperresponsiveness to diagnose asthma in New Zealand. Respir Med. 2006;100:2107–11.
46. Krouse JH. Asthma Management for the Otolaryngologist. Otolaryngol Clin N Am. 2017;50:1065–76.
47. Brigham EP, West NE. Diagnosis of asthma: diagnostic testing. Int Forum Allergy Rhinol. 2015;5(Suppl 1):S27–30.
48. Fokkens WJ, Lund VJ. Mullol jet al. EPOS 2012: European position paper on rhinosinusitis and nasal polyps 2012. A summary for otorhinolaryngologists. Rhinology. 2012;50:1–12.
49. Orlandi RR, Kingdom TT. Hwang PHet al. International consensus statement on allergy and rhinology: Rhinosinusitis. International forum of allergy & rhinology. 2016;6(Suppl 1):S22–209.
50. Staudacher AG, Stevens WW. Sinus infections, inflammation, and asthma. Immunol Allergy Clin N Am. 2019;39:403–15.
51. Jarvis D, Newson R. Lotvall jet al. Asthma in adults and its association with chronic rhinosinusitis: the GA2LEN survey in Europe. Allergy. 2012;67:91–8.
52. John Staniorski C, Price CPE. Weibman ARet al. Asthma onset pattern and patient outcomes in a chronic rhinosinusitis population. Int Forum Allergy Rhinol. 2018;8:495–503.
53. Batra PS, Tong L, Citardi MJ. Analysis of comorbidities and objective parameters in refractory chronic rhinosinusitis. Laryngoscope. 2013;123(Suppl 7):S1–11.
54. ten Brinke A, Grootendorst DC. Schmidt JTet al. Chronic sinusitis in severe asthma is related to sputum eosinophilia. J Allergy Clin Immunol. 2002;109:621–6.
55. Lin DC, Chandra RK. Tan BKet al. Association between severity of asthma and degree of chronic rhinosinusitis. Am J Rhinol Allergy. 2011;25:205–8.
56. ten Brinke A, Sterk PJ. Masclee AAet al. Risk factors of frequent exacerbations in difficult-to-treat asthma. Eur Respir J. 2005;26:812–8.
57. Tay TR, Radhakrishna N. Hore-Lacy Fet al. Comorbidities in difficult asthma are independent risk factors for frequent exacerbations, poor control and diminished quality of life. Respirology. 2016;21:1384–90.
58. Lee RU, Stevenson DD. Aspirin-exacerbated respiratory disease: evaluation and management. Allergy Asthma Immunol Res. 2011;3:3–10.

59. Stevens WW, Ocampo CJ. Berdnikovs set al. Cytokines in chronic Rhinosinusitis. Role in eosinophilia and aspirin-exacerbated respiratory disease. Am J Respir Crit Care Med. 2015;192:682–94.
60. Cahill KN, Bensko JC, Boyce JA, Laidlaw TM. Prostaglandin D(2): a dominant mediator of aspirin-exacerbated respiratory disease. J Allergy Clin Immunol. 2015;135:245–52.
61. Stevens WW, Peters AT, Hirsch AG, et al. Clinical Characteristics of Patients with Chronic Rhinosinusitis with Nasal Polyps, Asthma, and Aspirin-Exacerbated Respiratory Disease. J Allergy Clin Immunol Pract. 2017;5:1061–1070 e1063.
62. Jenkins C, Costello J, Hodge L. Systematic review of prevalence of aspirin induced asthma and its implications for clinical practice. BMJ. 2004;328:434.
63. Rajan JP, Wineinger NE, Stevenson DD, White AA. Prevalence of aspirin-exacerbated respiratory disease among asthmatic patients: a meta-analysis of the literature. J Allergy Clin Immunol. 2015;135:676–681 e671.
64. Ledford DK, Wenzel SE, Lockey RF. Aspirin or other nonsteroidal inflammatory agent exacerbated asthma. J Allergy Clin Immunol Pract. 2014;2:653–7.
65. Mascia K, Haselkorn T. Deniz YMet al. Aspirin sensitivity and severity of asthma: evidence for irreversible airway obstruction in patients with severe or difficult-to-treat asthma. J Allergy Clin Immunol. 2005;116:970–5.
66. Dursun AB, Woessner KA, Simon RA, Karasoy D, Stevenson DD. Predicting outcomes of oral aspirin challenges in patients with asthma, nasal polyps, and chronic sinusitis. Ann Allergy Asthma Immunol. 2008;100:420–5.
67. National Asthma E, Prevention P. Expert Panel Report 3 (EPR-3). Guidelines for the diagnosis and Management of Asthma-Summary Report 2007. J Allergy Clin Immunol. 2007;120:S94–138.
68. Pauwels RA, Pedersen S. Busse WWet al. Early intervention with budesonide in mild persistent asthma: a randomised, double-blind trial. Lancet. 2003;361:1071–6.
69. Adams NP, Bestall JB, Malouf R, Lasserson TJ, Jones PW. Inhaled beclomethasone versus placebo for chronic asthma. Cochrane Database Syst Rev. 2005:CD002738.
70. Drazen JM, Harrington D. New biologics for asthma. N Engl J Med. 2018;378:2533–4.
71. Hanania NA, Alpan O. Hamilos DLet al. Omalizumab in severe allergic asthma inadequately controlled with standard therapy: a randomized trial. Ann Intern Med. 2011;154:573–82.
72. Wenzel S, Ford L. Pearlman Det al. Dupilumab in persistent asthma with elevated eosinophil levels. N Engl J Med. 2013;368:2455–66.
73. Wang FP, Liu T, Lan Z, Li SY, Mao H. Efficacy and safety of anti-Interleukin-5 therapy in patients with asthma: a systematic review and meta-analysis. PLoS One. 2016;11:e0166833.
74. Snidvongs K, Kalish L, Sacks R, Craig JC, Harvey RJ. Topical steroid for chronic rhinosinusitis without polyps. Cochrane Database Syst Rev. 2011:CD009274.
75. Chong LY, Head K, Hopkins C, Philpott C, Schilder AG, Burton MJ. Intranasal steroids versus placebo or no intervention for chronic rhinosinusitis. Cochrane Database Syst Rev. 2016;(4):CD011996.
76. Kalish L, Snidvongs K, Sivasubramaniam R, Cope D, Harvey RJ. Topical steroids for nasal polyps. Cochrane Database Syst Rev. 2012;(12):CD006549.
77. American Lung Association-Asthma Clinical Research Centers' Writing C, Dixon AE. Castro met al. Efficacy of nasal mometasone for the treatment of chronic sinonasal disease in patients with inadequately controlled asthma. J Allergy Clin Immunol. 2015;135:701–709 e705.
78. Schaper C, Noga O. Koch bet al. Anti-inflammatory properties of montelukast, a leukotriene receptor antagonist in patients with asthma and nasal polyposis. J Investig Allergol Clin Immunol. 2011;21:51–8.
79. Ragab S, Parikh A, Darby YC, Scadding GK. An open audit of montelukast, a leukotriene receptor antagonist, in nasal polyposis associated with asthma. Clin Exp Allergy. 2001;31:1385–91.
80. Bachert C, Han JK. Desrosiers met al. Efficacy and safety of dupilumab in patients with severe chronic rhinosinusitis with nasal polyps (LIBERTY NP SINUS-24 and LIBERTY

NP SINUS-52): results from two multicentre, randomised, double-blind, placebo-controlled, parallel-group phase 3 trials. Lancet. 2019;394:1638–50.
81. Bachert C, Mannent L. Naclerio RMet al. Effect of subcutaneous Dupilumab on nasal polyp burden in patients with chronic sinusitis and nasal polyposis: a randomized clinical trial. JAMA. 2016;315:469–79.
82. Busse WW, Maspero JF. Rabe KFet al. Liberty asthma QUEST: phase 3 randomized, double-blind, placebo-controlled, parallel-group study to evaluate Dupilumab efficacy/safety in patients with uncontrolled, moderate-to-severe asthma. Adv Ther. 2018;35:737–48.
83. Simpson EL, Bieber T. Guttman-Yassky Eet al. Two phase 3 trials of Dupilumab versus placebo in atopic dermatitis. N Engl J Med. 2016;375:2335–48.
84. Lund VJ. The effect of sinonasal surgery on asthma. Allergy. 1999;54(Suppl 57):141–5.
85. Brown BL, Harner SG, Van Dellen RG. Nasal polypectomy in patients with asthma and sensitivity to aspirin. Arch Otolaryngol. 1979;105:413–6.
86. Moloney JR. Nasal polyps, nasal polypectomy, asthma, and aspirin sensitivity. Their association in 445 cases of nasal polyps. J Laryngol Otol. 1977;91:837–46.
87. Vashishta R, Soler ZM, Nguyen SA, Schlosser RJ. A systematic review and meta-analysis of asthma outcomes following endoscopic sinus surgery for chronic rhinosinusitis. Int Forum Allergy Rhinol. 2013;3:788–94.
88. Lee TJ, Fu CH. Wang CHet al. Impact of chronic rhinosinusitis on severe asthma patients. PLoS One. 2017;12:e0171047.
89. Schlosser RJ, Smith TL, Mace J, Soler ZM. Asthma quality of life and control after sinus surgery in patients with chronic rhinosinusitis. Allergy. 2017;72:483–91.
90. Chen FH, Zuo KJ. Guo YBet al. Long-term results of endoscopic sinus surgery-oriented treatment for chronic rhinosinusitis with asthma. Laryngoscope. 2014;124:24–8.
91. Hopkins C, Rimmer J, Lund VJ. Does time to endoscopic sinus surgery impact outcomes in chronic Rhinosinusitis? Prospective findings from the National Comparative Audit of surgery for nasal polyposis and chronic Rhinosinusitis. Rhinology. 2015;53:10–7.
92. Benninger MS, Sindwani R, Holy CE, Hopkins C. Impact of medically recalcitrant chronic rhinosinusitis on incidence of asthma. Int Forum Allergy Rhinol. 2016;6:124–9.
93. Dejima K, Hama T. Miyazaki met al. A clinical study of endoscopic sinus surgery for sinusitis in patients with bronchial asthma. Int Arch Allergy Immunol. 2005;138:97–104.
94. Rix I, Hakansson K, Larsen CG, Frendo M, von Buchwald C. Management of chronic rhinosinusitis with nasal polyps and coexisting asthma: a systematic review. Am J Rhinol Allergy. 2015;29:193–201.

Chapter 5
Asthma and Chronic Rhinosinusitis: Diagnosis and Medical Management

Daljit S. Mann, Sukaina Hasnie, and Kibwei A. McKinney

> **Key Concepts**
> - Systemic and topical steroids are common and effective medical treatment options for multiple phenotypes of asthma and CRS.
> - Monoclonal antibody biologic therapy targets specific components of the Th2-mediated inflammatory cascade and therefore can improve both sinonasal and pulmonary outcome measures.

In the second century, Claudius Galenus described the nose as a "respiratory instrument," a theory that has recently regained popularity. The airway, from the nose to the alveoli of the lungs, is described as a single functional unit in the unified airway theory [1]. Histologically, this theory is reflected by the common features of the respiratory epithelium that extends from the nasal septum and lateral nasal walls to the nasopharynx, larynx, trachea, bronchi, and bronchioles. The histologic characteristics include a pseudostratified columnar ciliated epithelium with goblet cells. Clinically, irritants from the environment, such as aeroallergens, microorganisms, and changes in inspired air, affect the mucosa of both the upper and lower airways [1]. This concept has brought into focus the connection between diseases of the upper and lower airways—specifically, the relationship between chronic rhinosinusitis (CRS) and asthma. Recent studies have expanded the understanding of lower airway diseases, including diagnostic considerations, management, treatment, and the quality of life of patients within the fields of otolaryngology, allergy and immunology, and pulmonology [2].

D. S. Mann · S. Hasnie · K. A. McKinney (✉)
Department of Otolaryngology – Head and Neck Surgery,
University of Oklahoma College of Medicine, Oklahoma City, OK, USA
e-mail: Kibwei-mckinney@ouhsc.edu

© Springer Nature Switzerland AG 2020
D. A. Gudis, R. J. Schlosser (eds.), *The Unified Airway*,
https://doi.org/10.1007/978-3-030-50330-7_5

Clinical Presentation

Asthma is a chronic condition that manifests with reversible and recurrent airway obstruction and bronchial hyperresponsiveness (BHR) secondary to inflammation of the lower airways [3]. The pathogenesis of asthma includes an antecedent exposure to a variety of irritants, including but not limited to tobacco smoke, pollutants, innumerable aeroallergens (such as ragweed, pollen, and animal dander), respiratory viral infections, and obesity [3].

The characteristic symptoms of asthma include wheezing, breathlessness, chest tightness, and coughing. This cough is typically dry and nonproductive and worsens at night or with increased levels of activity. The symptoms may vary in intensity but generally progress over time, resulting in morphological changes to the bronchial walls. Mild episodes are marked by symptoms that occur after physical activity, whereas severe episodes can occur even when patients are at rest. Children may present with drowsiness and confusion, at which point imminent respiratory distress should be suspected.

Rhinitis is characterized by irritation and inflammation of the upper airway mucosa that presents with sneezing, rhinorrhea, nasal congestion, and/or nasal itching. Rhinosinusitis is defined as inflammation of both the nasal mucosa and paranasal sinuses and presents with the above-listed symptoms in addition to sinus symptoms, which include facial pain and pressure, diminished sense of smell and taste, headaches, fatigue, and purulent anterior and/or posterior nasal drainage. Patients may have rhinitis without sinusitis. Chronic rhinosinusitis is defined as symptomatic rhinosinusitis lasting greater than 12 weeks in duration.

Demographic Considerations

It is estimated that asthma affects over 300 million individuals worldwide. The Center of Disease Control and Prevention (CDC) reports that currently 8.4% of children and 8.1% of adults in the United States are affected by asthma [2]. It is the most common chronic childhood illness, accounting for 13.8 million missed school days and 1.3 million emergency room visits annually. Women tend to have a higher prevalence than men, with a ratio of 9.9:7.0. There is also a higher death rate among women and non-Hispanic blacks when compared with other groups [2].

CRS is estimated to have a prevalence of 10%–12% in the general population and is estimated to affect nearly 50 million individuals every year. In the United States, 146 per 1000 persons are suspected to be suffering from CRS, with an increasing incidence every year. CRS is responsible for 18–22 million physician visits per year in the United States alone, with a direct treatment cost of $3.4–5 billion annually [4]. Currently, CRS is the fifth most common disease to be treated with antibiotics.

Multiple studies have been conducted to investigate the merits of the unified airway theory. In 1991, Annesi-Maesano et al. reported the concordance rate of CRS and asthma to be 34% [5]. Gene interactions have also been found to contribute to the development of asthma in several studies. A study conducted in Northern Sweden found that a family history of asthma or rhinitis is associated with a three- to four-fold increased risk for the development of adult onset asthma and a two- to six-fold increased risk of developing rhinitis, when compared to those without a family history [2].

Phenotypes

A number of different phenotypes have been proposed for the classification of asthma based on distinguishing factors such as the type of trigger, age of onset, and clinical presentation. The most common classification differentiates asthma into two broad categories on the basis of the frequency of symptoms: intermittent asthma and persistent asthma. The persistent domain contains the following subtypes: mild persistent, moderate persistent, and severe persistent from the 2007 National Asthma Education and Prevention Program (NAEPP) guidelines (Fig. 5.1). More recently, in 2019, the Global Initiative for Asthma (GINA) redefined severity according to the level of treatment required to control symptoms (Fig. 5.2). The GINA 2019 guidelines stressed a difference between severe and uncontrolled asthma, suggesting that controlling external factors may resolve uncontrolled asthma. CRS is now listed and recognized as a comorbidity and complicating condition that may contribute to uncontrolled asthma.

The two most common phenotypes of CRS in the literature are chronic rhinosinusitis with nasal polyps (CRSwNP) and chronic rhinosinusitis without nasal polyps (CRSsNP). Multiple studies have found that CRSwNP is associated with more severe asthma. The National Heart, Lung, and Blood Institute's Severe Asthma Research Program (SARP) analyzed patients in clusters of the age of onset and lung severity and found that late-onset asthmatics had a higher frequency of sinus disease, radiographic changes, and rates of sinus surgery [3].

CRSwNP however has been found to cluster into many different phenotypes based on underlying pathogenic mechanisms. Dennis et al. established four classification methods for endotyping patients with CRSwNP [6]. The first approach is the type 2 cytokine-based schema, in which CRSwNP is differentiated based on the upregulation of Type 1 versus Type 2 pathways. The second approach focuses on the aberrant Th2 pathway, differentiating CRS subtypes based on the presence of an eosinophilic versus neutrophilic mucosal infiltrates. Eosinophilic chronic rhinosinusitis (eCRS) has been found to display a severe medically and surgically refractory clinical course when compared to non-eCRS subtypes. The third schema classifies subtypes of CRS based on different levels of IgE, which is elevated in all cases of CRSwNP except in some cases of aspirin-exacerbated respiratory disease (AERD). Lastly, AERD versus non-AERD disease differentiates CRS subtypes according to a cysteinyl leukotriene (CysLT)-based approach [6].

AERD, a hypersensitivity reaction to acetylsalicylic acid and cyclooxygenase (COX)-1-inhibiting nonsteroidal anti-inflammatory drugs, is considered not only a phenotype of CRSwNP but also a subtype of asthma [7]. AERD presents with

INITIAL VISIT: CLASSIFYING ASTHMA SEVERITY AND INITIATING THERAPY

(in patients who are not currently taking long-term control medications)

Level of severity (Columns 2–5) is determined by events listed in Column 1 for both impairment (frequency and intensity of symptoms and functional limitations) and risk (of exacerbations). Assess impairment by patient's or caregiver's recall of events during the previous 2–4 weeks; assess risk over the last year. Recommendations for initiating therapy based on level of severity are presented in the last row.

	Components of Severity	Intermittent			Persistent: Mild			Persistent: Moderate			Persistent: Severe		
		Ages 0–4 years	Ages 5–11 years	Ages ≥12 years	Ages 0–4 years	Ages 5–11 years	Ages ≥12 years	Ages 0–4 years	Ages 5–11 years	Ages ≥12 years	Ages 0–4 years	Ages 5–11 years	Ages ≥12 years
Impairment	Symptoms	≤2 days/week			>2 days/week but not daily			Daily			Throughout the day		
	Nighttime awakenings	0	≤2x/month		1–2x/month	3–4x/month		3–4x/month	>1x/week but not nightly		>1x/week	Often 7x/week	
	SABA* use for symptom control (not to prevent EIB*)	≤2 days/week			>2 days/week but not daily	>2 days/week but not daily and not more than once on any day		Daily			Several times per day		
	Interference with normal activity	None			Minor limitation			Some limitation			Extremely limited		
	Lung function		Normal FEV_1 between exacerbations	Normal FEV_1 between exacerbations									
	➔ FEV_1* (% predicted)	Not applicable	>80%	>80%	Not applicable	>80%	>80%	Not applicable	60–80%	60–80%	Not applicable	<60%	<60%
	➔ FEV_1/FVC *		>85%	Normal †		>80%	Normal †		75–80%	Reduced 5% †		<75%	Reduced >5% †
Risk	Asthma exacerbations requiring oral systemic corticosteroids ‡	0–1/year			≥2 exacerb. in 6 months, or wheezing ≥4x per year lasting >1 day AND risk factors for persistent asthma	Generally, more frequent and intense events indicate greater severity.							
						≥2/year	Generally, more frequent and intense events indicate greater severity.						
		Consider severity and interval since last asthma exacerbation. Frequency and severity may fluctuate over time for patients in any severity category. Relative annual risk of exacerbations may be related to FEV_1.*											
	Recommended Step for Initiating Therapy (See "Stepwise Approach for Managing Asthma Long Term," page 7) The stepwise approach is meant to help, not replace, the clinical decisionmaking needed to meet individual patient needs.	Step 1			Step 2			Step 3	Step 3 medium-dose ICS* option	Step 3	Step 3	Step 3 medium-dose ICS* option or Step 4	Step 4 or 5
								Consider short course of oral systemic corticosteroids.					
		In 2–6 weeks, depending on severity, assess level of asthma control achieved and adjust therapy as needed. For children 0–4 years old, if no clear benefit is observed in 4–6 weeks, consider adjusting therapy or alternate diagnoses.											

* **Abbreviations:** EIB, exercise-induced bronchospasm; FEV_1, forced expiratory volume in 1 second; FVC, forced vital capacity; ICS, inhaled corticosteroid; SABA, short-acting $beta_2$-agonist.

† Normal FEV_1/FVC by age: 8–19 years, 85%; 20–39 years, 80%; 40–59 years, 75%; 60–80 years, 70%.

‡ Data are insufficient to link frequencies of exacerbations with different levels of asthma severity. Generally, more frequent and intense exacerbations (e.g., requiring urgent care, hospital or intensive care admission, and/or oral corticosteroids) indicate greater underlying disease severity. For treatment purposes, patients with ≥2 exacerbations may be considered to have persistent asthma, even in the absence of impairment levels consistent with persistent asthma.

Asthma Care Quick Reference ■ 5

Fig. 5.1 Classifying asthma severity and initiating treatment. Level of severity (Columns 2–5) is determined by events listed in Column 1 for both impairment (frequency and intensity of symptoms and functional limitations) and risk (of exacerbations). Assess impairment by patient's or caregiver's recall of events during the previous 2–4 weeks; assess risk over the last year. Recommendations for initiating therapy based on the level of severity are presented in the last row. Abbreviations: EIB, exercise-induced bronchospasm; FEV1, forced expiratory volume in 1 second; FVC, forced vital capacity; ICS, inhaled corticosteroid; SABA, short-acting beta2-agonist. † Normal FEV1/FVC by age: 8–19 years, 85%; 20–39 years, 80%; 40–59 years, 75%; 60–80 years, 70%. ‡ Data are insufficient to link frequencies of exacerbations with different levels of asthma severity. Generally, more frequent and intense exacerbations (e.g., requiring urgent care, hospital or intensive care admission, and/or oral corticosteroids) indicate greater underlying disease severity. For treatment purposes, patients with ≥2 exacerbations may be considered to have persistent asthma, even in the absence of impairment levels consistent with persistent asthma. (From National Heart, Lung, and Blood Institute; National Institutes of Health; U.S. Department of Health and Human Services. https://www.nhlbi.nih.gov/sites/default/files/media/docs/12-5075.pdf)

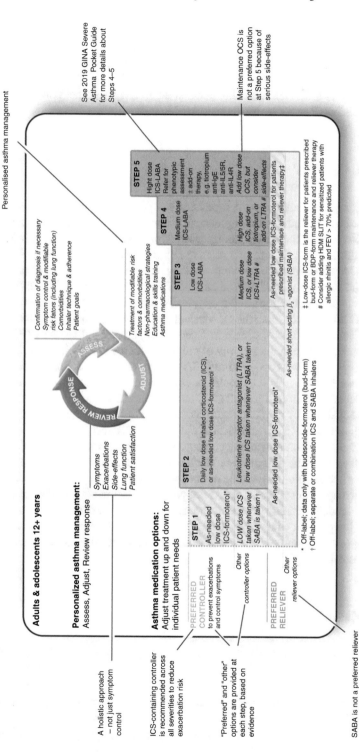

Fig. 5.2 GINA 2019. (From Pocket Guide for Asthma Management and Prevention: (for Adults and Children Older than 5 Years) Global Initiative for Asthma, 2018, with permission)

overexpression of CysLT as a result of defective COX enzymes and increased activity of the 5-lipoxygenase and leukotriene C4 synthase pathways. It usually presents in the second decade of life, affecting both the upper and lower airways. AERD prevalence in the general adult asthmatic population is 7%, while in severe asthmatic patients, it is 14%. Dennis et al. noted that the frequency of the AERD phenotype within CRSwNP is approximately 10% [6].

Diagnostic Criteria

Asthma is a diagnosis based on a comprehensive evaluation of the subjective and objective findings, including a comprehensive history and physical examination in combination with pulmonary function tests. A positive family history has been found to confer a 6.7-fold increased relative risk and thus should be investigated thoroughly. Other risk factors including smoking, environmental irritant exposure, and other signs of atopy should also be queried. PFTs are considered the gold standard for the diagnosis of asthma and are typically conducted with the use of a spirometer. PFTs must demonstrate the presence of airway obstruction, as indicated by a decreased forced-expiratory-volume-in-1-second-to-forced-vital-capacity (FEV1/FVC) ratio and a change in the severity of the obstruction when subjected to bronchodilatory or bronchoconstrictive stimuli. The change should be defined as at least a 20% increase in the FEV1. It should be considered that PFTs may be normal during clinical examination in patients without an acute flare. Such patients should have a bronchopulmonary challenge with repeat PFTs to confirm the diagnosis.

The diagnosis of CRS is established with the persistence of symptoms for 12 weeks or longer in duration and documented evidence of inflammation [8]. Two or more of the following symptoms must be present: anterior or posterior nasal drainage, nasal obstruction, hyposmia or anosmia, and/or facial pain and pressure. Inflammation may be documented by at least one of the following: purulent mucus, edema of the middle meatus, polyps in the nasal cavity or middle meatus, and/or radiographic imaging showing inflammation of the paranasal sinuses [8]. A focused sinonasal history and thorough physical exam including nasal endoscopy should therefore be obtained.

Physical Examination

Physical examination in asthma should consist of an evaluation of the patient's vital signs, auscultation of the chest, and a survey for the signs of respiratory distress, including the use of accessory muscles of respiration. Patients experiencing a severe asthma episode typically present with breathlessness at rest, a respiratory rate greater than 30 breaths per minute, suprasternal retractions, a heart rate greater than 120 bpm, and auscultation of loud biphasic expiratory and inspiratory wheezing.

Physical examination for CRS should include anterior rhinoscopy, which may reveal the presence of purulent nasal drainage, nasal obstruction, polyposis, and inflammation of the nasal mucosa. If anterior rhinoscopy is unrevealing or a more detailed examination is warranted, a formal nasal endoscopy is warranted.

Laboratory Testing

While not conducted often, mucosal swabs and biopsies have revealed similar cellular infiltrates in both CRS and asthma, including the presence of eosinophils, mast cells, macrophages, and T cells. Patients in whom allergic asthma is suspected may undergo skin testing and in vitro ImmunoCAP IgE testing. Recent research efforts have focused on biomarker analysis for the identification of phenotypes that may delineate endotype-specific treatment algorithms and improved management outcomes. Nitric oxide (FeNO), serum IgE, sputum and blood eosinophil count, and serum periostin comprise some of the biomarkers currently being studied in the asthma population [2]. For CRS, the evaluation of IL-5 levels has been increasingly investigated, due to the availability of anti-IL5 monoclonal antibodies. Other markers that have garnered interest include epithelial-derived cytokines (IL-25 and IL-33), type 2 innate lymphoid cells (ILC2s), IL-4, IL-13, and, in the setting of AERD, urinary leukotriene C4.

Radiographic Imaging

Chest radiography is most commonly used in the workup of asthma. The main purpose of the chest X-ray is to rule out other causes of reactive airway disease that may present with similar symptoms. Patients with asthma typically have normal chest X-ray but may occasionally display hyperinflation of the lung fields.

Plain films are no longer used to diagnose CRS, due to their limited diagnostic value. Noncontrast computed tomography (CT) scans have now become the gold-standard imaging modality for the diagnosis of CRS. CT scans have the ability to detect mucosal disease and anatomical pathology within the sinuses that are not visible via endoscopy, including the presence of sinonasal polyps, mucous membrane thickening, and ostiomeatal obstruction. The Lund-Mackay scoring system is a 24-point grading schema that assesses 6 anatomical regions on each side of the nose on a scale from 0 to 2. A score of 0 correlates to the absence of disease, 1 indicates partial opacification, and 2 demonstrates complete opacification of each anatomical area. These scores have been found to provide relevant data on location and extent of disease; however, they do not always predict or correlate with patient symptoms. The posterior ethmoid sinus and olfactory cleft have been found to be the anatomical regions that are most predictive of subjective symptoms. However, it should be noted that a sinus CT should only be ordered if the patient has at least two of the above-listed symptomatic complaints, due to high false-positive rates.

A number of reviews have been performed previously that demonstrate evidence of mucous membrane thickening in patients with asthma who do not have a documented history of CRS [9, 10]. One study conducted recently found that in patients with severe asthma, sputum eosinophilia and positive pulmonary function tests correlated with abnormal sinus CT changes [5].

Sinonasal Endoscopy

Endoscopic evaluation of CRS is routinely performed and may reveal mucopurulence, mucosal edema, and sinonasal polyposis. Nasal endoscopy can help to detect any anatomical abnormalities or sinus disease that may affect mucociliary clearance and airway patency. Many studies have been conducted to evaluate the effect of sinonasal endoscopy in the diagnosis of CRS relative to accepted imaging modalities. Bhattacharyya and Lee found that endoscopy, paired with the symptom criteria as designated by the American Academy of Otolaryngology-Head and Neck Surgery (AAO-HNS) guidelines, improved diagnostic accuracy and odds ratio by 26.3% and 3.5%, respectively, when compared to CT [7].

Several studies have also proposed the routine use of sinonasal endoscopy in patients with asthma in order to diagnose unrecognized CRS. For example, Ameli et al. found purulent rhinosinusitis in 47.6% of asthmatic children in their study population [11]. Feng et al. similarly found a significant correlation between nasal endoscopy score and the duration of asthma, suggesting that examination of the nasal airway should be a part of standard clinical assessment of patients with asthma [12].

Quality of Life Questionnaires

Recent data reveals that while diagnostic measures such as pulmonary function tests, radiographic imaging, and endoscopic evaluation are key for the diagnosis of CRS and asthma, questionnaires of subjective symptoms should be conducted to evaluate symptoms and disease severity. The merits of this approach are unclear, as the subjective metrics of disease severity reported by patients do not always match the objective findings of the clinical evaluation.

Many validated, disease-specific symptom surveys have been developed for CRS including the Sino-Nasal Outcome Test-22 (SNOT-22), Rhinoconjunctivitis Quality of Life Questionnaire (RQLQ), Nasal symptom score (NSS), and rhinosinusitis disability index (RSDI). For asthma, the Asthma Control Test (ACT) is most frequently used. The ACT evaluates the control of asthmatic symptoms through the following five items: activity limitations, shortness of breath, nighttime waking, the frequency of use of asthma relief medications, and complications that are the direct result of asthma symptoms. A recent study utilized these questionnaires to evaluate the symptoms of patients with concordant asthma and CRS with failed medical treatment before and after sinus surgery [1]. The study found that severe sinonasal symptoms of CRS were associated with poorly controlled asthma and that nasal surgery improved not only sinonasal symptoms but also asthma control and PFT results. Even in this case, the accuracy of self-reported symptoms had low sensitivity (84%) and specificity (82%) for predicting CRS.

Medical Management and Outcomes

Given the robust association between asthma and CRS, the question is raised about whether the treatment of one disease has an impact on the control of the other pathologic process. Medical therapies including saline irrigation, intranasal and systemic glucocorticoids, antibiotics, and anti-leukotriene agents are used in the treatment of CRS with and without nasal polyposis. Medications for asthma are broadly categorized as long-term control medications, used to achieve and maintain control of persistent asthma, or relieving medications, used to treat acute symptoms and exacerbations. The mainstay of medical therapy for asthma includes inhaled corticosteroids, long- and short-acting beta-2 agonists, anti-leukotriene agents, muscarinic antagonists, and biologic therapy.

Topical Medical Therapy: Intranasal Steroids

Intranasal corticosteroids are recommended and widely accepted for the treatment of CRS as inflammation is considered to be the pathologic basis for the disease. There are several systematic reviews that support topical steroid therapy for the treatment of CRS with polyposis [13, 14], and it is reflected in the clinical practice guidelines for the treatment of adult sinusitis [8].

First-generation intranasal steroids include beclomethasone, triamcinolone, flunisolide, and budesonide. Second-generation agents include fluticasone, mometasone, and ciclesonide. A Cochrane systematic review published in 2016 compared first- and second-generation medications, as well as high versus low steroid dosing. There was minimal and low-quality evidence that did not reveal any significant difference in efficacy between the available options. High and low dosing of intranasal steroids was also found to have similar efficacy; however, the lower dose was associated with fewer side effects and episodes of epistaxis [13].

There is scarce data analyzing the effects of intranasal steroid use and the subsequent effect on asthma control. A multicenter placebo-controlled 24-week trial of nasal mometasone in patients with CRS and poorly controlled asthma showed no benefit for asthma control in children or adults [15]. This suggests that the treatment of CRS alone with corticosteroids is not efficacious in improving asthma outcomes. Treatment with intranasal steroids should therefore remain targeted to the symptoms of rhinosinusitis and allergic rhinitis [15]. A meta-analysis by Lohia et al. also demonstrated that the use of intranasal corticosteroid medications is associated with the improvement of asthma-specific outcome measures in patients suffering from both allergic rhinitis and asthma [16].

Systemic Medical Therapy

Steroids

Oral steroids are most often used in patients with chronic rhinosinusitis with nasal polyposis. Short courses of steroids (14–21 days) are typically prescribed in an attempt to limit inflammation within the nasal cavity, reduce the burden of sinonasal polyps, and improve nasal symptoms. A Cochrane review and meta-analysis of eight randomized-control studies compared the effect of a short course of systemic steroid treatment with placebo or no treatment [17]. Oral steroid regimens included in the review used prednisone, prednisolone, and methylprednisolone, with varying doses. The findings indicate that there is an improvement in disease-specific health-related quality of life [18, 19] and nasal polyp burden [19, 20] immediately after treatment is completed. However, when these outcomes were compared at 3–6 months after treatment, nasal polyp scores and quality-of-life outcomes were not significantly different between the two study arms [19]. Bulbul et al. also studied the effects of combined oral steroids as an adjunct to intranasal steroids. When compared to receiving intranasal steroids alone, the authors demonstrated an improvement in mean nasal polyp size after a 21-day treatment course [21].

In patients with asthma, oral steroids are prescribed to help control symptoms in the case of an acute asthma exacerbation that requires emergency room evaluation. They have been shown to reduce the rate of repeat exacerbation [22]. Optimal dosing of oral steroids for acute asthma exacerbation remains unknown; however, a systematic review sought to identify the optimal dosing and duration [23]. The review included 18 studies that compared prednisolone and dexamethasone at different doses and durations, but did not yield convincing evidence of any difference in outcomes. The current guidelines set by the Global Initiative for Asthma recommend a dosing equivalent of prednisolone 50 mg daily for a course of 5–7 days [24].

To date, there is no available literature that evaluates the effects of a given steroid course on the unified airway. However, because oral steroids are prescribed for CRS in a similar manner to courses given for asthma exacerbations, future studies should be designed to study the treatment effect on both systems.

Anti-Leukotrienes

Anti-leukotriene drugs are classified based on the mechanism of action as either leukotriene receptor antagonists (LTRA) or leukotriene synthesis inhibitors [25]. LTRAs (zafirlukast, pranlukast, montelukast) block the leukotriene receptor and the end-organ response of the pathway. Leukotriene synthesis inhibitors (zileuton) are 5-lipoxygenase inhibitors that block the synthesis of leukotrienes [25].

In the management of asthma, anti-leukotrienes are not as effective as inhaled corticosteroids as a monotherapeutic agent [26]. In patients with poor asthma control with moderate to severe symptoms, using LTRAs as an adjunct to inhaled corticosteroids has been shown to reduce asthma exacerbations and improve lung function [27].

In patients with CRS with nasal polyposis, studies have shown increased levels of eosinophilic inflammatory markers, leukotrienes, and leukotriene receptors that localize to nasal polyps [28, 29]. Montelukast has been shown to improve the severity of symptoms as well as objective clinical measurements such as polyp size and immune profiles of patients with CRSwNP when compared to placebo [25, 30]. A systematic review by Wentzel et al. identified several case series and RCTs that assessed the treatment effect on patients with asthma and CRS; however, there were no differences in the objective or subjective outcomes of CRS based on asthma status [30].

Antibiotics

There is no definitive role for the use of antibiotics in the treatment of chronic rhinosinusitis. The 2015 clinical practice guidelines from the American Academy of Otolaryngology-Head and Neck Surgery discuss the role of several antibiotic classes in treating acute bacterial rhinosinusitis (ABRS) but do not mention their role in treating CRS, as it largely remains unclear. Selection of antibiotic use in acute versus chronic rhinosinusitis is also very different. In ARS/ABRS, empiric antibiotic selection is based on the microbiome and the prevalence of common pathogens [8]. As CRS is now considered to be an inflammatory disease state, most antibiotic regimens include macrolides or doxycycline because of their anti-inflammatory properties. There is some evidence that a short course (3 weeks) of doxycycline may lead to a decrease in polyp burden [31], but there is limited data on the use of long-term antibiotics. A 2016 Cochrane review by Head et al. included four RCTs that compared oral antibiotics to placebo, with a minimum follow up of 3 months. The authors concluded that there is very little evidence that systemic antibiotics are effective in treating CRS. There is some evidence that an oral macrolide may improve disease-specific quality of life in CRS patients without polyposis at the end of a 3-month treatment course [32]. A more recently published review by Barshak et al. included two additional RCTs [33, 34] and came to similar conclusions [35].

Similarly for asthma, macrolide therapy has been studied for its long-term anti-inflammatory effects and for control of the intracellular infections *Chlamydophila pneumoniae* or *Mycoplasma pneumoniae* [36, 37]. A 2015 Cochrane review of 23 studies, for a total of 1513 participants, included patients randomized to receive macrolide or placebo [38]. Treatment with macrolides was not found to confer any benefit over placebo for the majority of outcomes assessed, including exacerbations, frequency of treatment with oral steroids, quality of life, and rescue medication use. There was some evidence that macrolides led to some improvement in symptom scales and in lung function (FEV_1) [38] and may have a steroid-sparing effect [38–40]. Among these studies, there is significant variation in macrolide choice, dosage, frequency, and duration of treatment which leads to low-quality evidence to support their use. A more recently published review and meta-analysis of the effects of azithromycin in asthma by Wang et al. revealed similar improvement in FEV_1 without evidence of improvement in clinical outcomes such as the frequency of asthma exacerbations and quality-of-life outcomes [41].

Immunotherapy

Allergen-specific immunotherapy has been shown to be efficacious in improving symptoms and reducing medication use in allergic asthma by altering the immune response to allergens [42, 43]. Immunotherapy is also beneficial when allergic asthma and rhinitis are concurrent [42, 44]. Subcutaneous (SCIT) and sublingual (SLIT) immunotherapy are the two main routes of administration. SCIT has been shown to reduce the development of asthma in children with allergic rhinitis [45], and follow up studies have confirmed that the long-term preventative effects of asthma were sustained up to 7 years after cessation of therapy [46]. SLIT with grass pollen tablets in patients with allergic rhinitis has also been shown to be associated with fewer asthma diagnoses, slower progression of the disease, and a decrease in medication use after completion of SLIT [47]. For adult patients with sensitivity to house dust mite, SLIT has also been shown to help decrease mild to moderate asthma exacerbations [48].

Biologic Agents

Biologic therapy targets specific immune cells and cytokines within the inflammatory cascade to control the underlying inflammation. Several therapies have been approved for patients with severe asthma [49]. With the overlap in the pathophysiology of asthma and CRSwNP, patients with concurrent disease were found to have improvements in both sinonasal and asthma symptoms [50]. Current trials for biologic therapies in CRS have therefore focused on patients with nasal polyposis and the Th2-mediated inflammatory pathway [51]. The majority of the biologic drugs under investigation have not been examined in CRS patients; however, there are five that have been studied for use in patients with CRSwNP: omalizumab, mepolizumab, reslizumab, benralizumab, and dupilumab [51].

Omalizumab is an anti-IgE monoclonal antibody that has been approved for use in moderate to severe uncontrolled asthma and has also been shown to improve polyp size and sinonasal symptoms [52]. In patients with comorbid CRSwNP and severe asthma undergoing omalizumab treatment, a recent study has shown a reduction in the rates of antibiotic prescriptions after treatment, as well as a reduction of oral steroid use during treatment [53].

Reslizumab and mepolizumab are monoclonal antibodies that target IL-5, which stimulates eosinophil activation. Both drugs are currently in clinical trials and have demonstrated a significant reduction in polyp size but did not show significant symptomatic improvement [54]. Benralizumab targets the IL-5 receptor and has completed phase 3 trials for eosinophilic asthma which showed improvement in lung function, asthma symptoms, and reduction in exacerbations [55]. The drug is still being studied for its effects on CRS, and results have yet to be published [51].

Dupilumab is a monoclonal antibody to the α subunit of the IL-4 receptor which inhibits signaling of both IL-4 and IL-13 cytokines [51]. Bachert et al. demonstrated improvements in polyp size, disease-specific quality of life, and olfactory function [56].

Case Report

A 16-year-old female presented with a history of chronic rhinosinusitis, allergic rhinitis, eczema, and asthma of 7 years in duration. Her presenting symptoms included nasal obstruction; thick, clear rhinorrhea; facial pain and pressure; purulent posterior nasal drainage; and headaches. Her respiratory symptoms included recurrent exacerbations that were marked by wheezing, chest tightness, and difficulty lying supine. The patient had frequently visited the emergency department due to this constellation of symptoms. Her atopic disease was being managed with albuterol, omeprazole, cetirizine, and fluticasone/salmeterol. She also underwent allergy testing, which revealed multiple systemic hypersensitivities 2 years prior to presentation and was receiving subcutaneous immunotherapy, with no significant clinical improvement in her allergic or atopic symptoms.

Initially, an attempt was made to optimize her medical management with the addition of daily sinus rinses, intranasal fluticasone, and systemic steroids and antibiotics as needed, for acute flares. Despite these changes to her treatment regimen, she was noted to have recalcitrant sinonasal polyposis on follow-up sinonasal endoscopy, without any symptomatic relief. A posttreatment CT scan of the sinuses was obtained that corroborated these findings, including obstruction of the frontal and spheno-ethmoidal recesses and partial opacification of the ethmoid and maxillary sinuses (Figs. 5.3 and 5.4). Based on these recalcitrant findings, functional endoscopic sinus surgery was performed, including bilateral maxillary antrostomies, total sphenoethmoidectomies, and frontal sinusotomies. Intraoperative findings included severe polyposis in the bilateral maxillary sinuses and moderate polyposis within the bilateral sphenoid, ethmoid, and frontal sinuses.

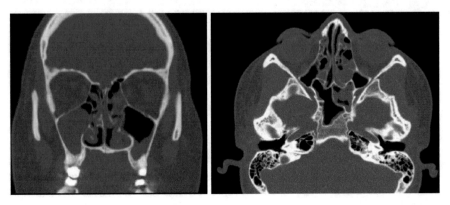

Fig. 5.3 Coronal and axial views of noncontrast CT sinus, obtained preoperatively, following a course of appropriate medical therapy. There is significant mucous membrane thickening in the bilateral ethmoid and maxillary sinuses, with near-total opacification of the right maxillary sinus

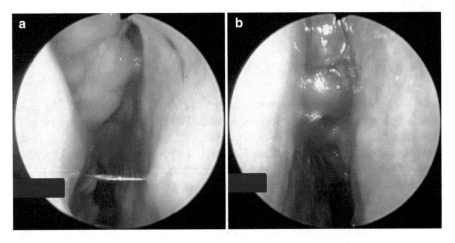

Fig. 5.4 (**a, b**) Preoperative sinonasal endoscopy of the right and left middle meatuses. There is extensive polyp overgrowth extending beyond the lower edge of the middle turbinate

Initially, the patient did well, with the improvement of her nasal obstruction and resolution of her facial pain and pressure. Unfortunately, 1 month postoperatively, the patient's symptoms returned with endoscopic evidence of polyp regrowth and mucopurulent drainage. Cultures were obtained that demonstrated growth of methicillin-resistant *Staphylococcus aureus* (MRSA). She was treated with courses of oral prednisone and culture-directed trimethoprim-sulfamethoxazole and started on topical budesonide nasal irrigations. During follow-up in postoperative months 2 and 3, she had persistent symptoms of nasal obstruction, facial pain, and purulent discharge. Sinonasal endoscopy revealed significant bilateral crusting with mucopurulent drainage and polyp regrowth in the bilateral maxillary sinuses and along the ethmoid skull base. Repeat imaging during postoperative month 3 also revealed persistent disease, as seen in Fig. 5.5. Given the persistence of symptoms and recurrent

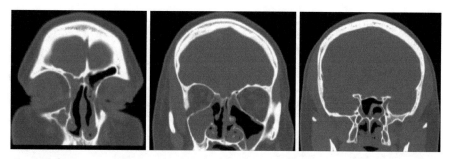

Fig. 5.5 Postoperative noncontrast CT scan of the sinuses, following culture-directed antibiotics which were initiated for the recalcitrant disease. This demonstrates opacification of the bilateral maxillary sinuses and right frontal recess, with lateralization and polypoid degeneration of the middle turbinates

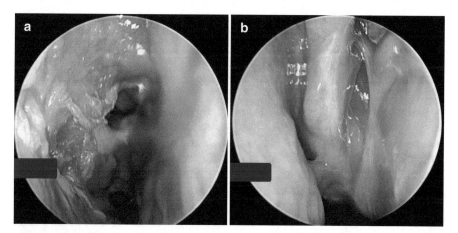

Fig. 5.6 (a, b) Sinonasal endoscopy 3 months postoperatively following revision sinus surgery and bilateral resection of the middle turbinates. This demonstrates mucopurulent drainage emanating from the middle meatus and cicatricial stenosis of the sphenoid ostium

disease, the patient was taken back for revision surgery 4 months postoperatively. At that time, the bilateral middle turbinates were truncated due to extensive polypoid degeneration and destabilization, in order to allow for improved delivery of topical treatments to the middle meatus.

One month following revision surgery, she had recurrent nasal congestion, facial pressure, and yellow purulent drainage. Directed sinus culture revealed MRSA infection that was sensitive to gentamycin. At that juncture, the patient was started on a 2-month course of topical gentamycin rinses with baby shampoo to help with the crusting and persistent infection. Diluted baby shampoo nasal irrigations have been shown to help improve symptoms of thickened nasal discharge, crusting, and postnasal drainage in the postoperative patient [57]. Three months postoperatively, the topical treatment had helped to improve her purulent drainage and obstructive symptoms, although she had some continued crusting and polyposis along the bilateral ethmoid skull base as seen in Fig. 5.6. She was also experiencing worsening of

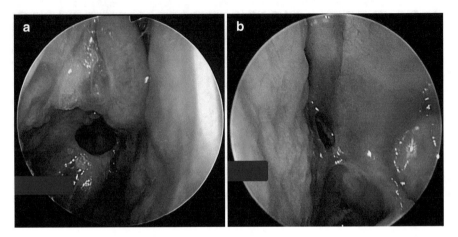

Fig. 5.7 (**a, b**) Sinonasal endoscopy 3 months after the initiation of treatment with dupilumab. The burden of sinonasal polyposis has diminished significantly and the maxillary and sphenoid ostia remain widely patent

her asthma and atopic dermatitis, and the biologic dupilumab was initiated by the patient's pulmonologist.

One month after the initiation of dupilumab, the patient reported a significant improvement in nasal obstruction, posterior nasal drainage, and facial pain and pressure. In addition, her atopic dermatitis, which included extensive pruritis, papules, and xerosis of the facial skin, completely resolved. Her asthma symptoms similarly improved, and she was able to discontinue the use of her rescue inhaler. Sinonasal endoscopy revealed resolution of mucosal inflammation of the ethmoid, sphenoid, and maxillary sinuses and only mild crusting in the right maxillary sinus and nonobstructive polyposis along the ethmoid skull base (Fig. 5.7).

Conclusion

The unified airway theory helps to explain the interdependence of the signs, symptoms, and severity of CRS and asthma. This relationship is being actively studied in patients with concomitant diagnoses in order to better understand these disease processes. Accurate assessment and diagnosis is necessary in order to identify and improve the severity of symptoms and the quality of life of patients with this phenotype. Previously, management has been aimed at improving each disease process as a separate entity. With a growing understanding of the interrelatedness of these diseases, novel biologic agents are being developed that target the pathophysiologic inflammatory pathways that are common to each. These agents show promise in treating patients with concurrent disease.

References

1. Huang C-C, Wang C-H, Fu C-H, et al. The link between chronic rhinosinusitis and asthma: a questionnaire-based study. Medicine (Baltimore). 2016;95(31):e4294. https://doi.org/10.1097/MD.0000000000004294.

2. Massoth L, Anderson C, McKinney KA. Asthma and chronic rhinosinusitis: diagnosis and medical management. Med Sci (Basel, Switzerland). 2019;7(4). https://doi.org/10.3390/medsci7040053.

3. Dougherty RH, Fahy JV. Acute exacerbations of asthma: epidemiology, biology and the exacerbation-prone phenotype. Clin Exp Allergy J Br Soc Allergy Clin Immunol. 2009;39(2):193–202. https://doi.org/10.1111/j.1365-2222.2008.03157.x.

4. Pleis JR, Lucas JW. Summary health statistics for U.S. adults: National Health Interview Survey, 2007. Vital Health Stat. 2009;10(240):1–159.

5. ten Brinke A, Grootendorst DC, Schmidt JT, et al. Chronic sinusitis in severe asthma is related to sputum eosinophilia. J Allergy Clin Immunol. 2002;109(4):621–6. https://doi.org/10.1067/mai.2002.122458.

6. Dennis SK, Lam K, Luong A. A review of classification schemes for chronic rhinosinusitis with nasal polyposis endotypes. Laryngoscope Investig Otolaryngol. 2016;1(5):130–4. https://doi.org/10.1002/lio2.32.

7. Deosthale NV, Khadakkar SP, Harkare VV, et al. Diagnostic accuracy of nasal endoscopy as compared to computed tomography in chronic rhinosinusitis. Indian J Otolaryngol Head Neck Surg. 2017;69(4):494–9. https://doi.org/10.1007/s12070-017-1232-0.

8. Rosenfeld RM, Piccirillo JF, Chandrasekhar SS, et al. Clinical practice guideline (Update): adult sinusitis. 2015. https://doi.org/10.1177/0194599815572097.

9. Hansen AG, Helvik A-S, Thorstensen WM, et al. Paranasal sinus opacification at MRI in lower airway disease (the HUNT study-MRI). Eur Arch Otorhinolaryngol. 2016;273(7):1761–8. https://doi.org/10.1007/s00405-015-3790-7.

10. Adapinar B, Kurt E, Kebapçi M, Erginel MS. Computed tomography evaluation of paranasal sinuses in asthma: is there a tendency of particular site involvement? Allergy Asthma Proc. 2006;27(6):504–9. https://doi.org/10.2500/aap.2006.27.2892.

11. Ameli F, Castelnuovo P, Pagella F, et al. Nasal endoscopy in asthmatic children: clinical role in the diagnosis of rhinosinusitis. Rhinology. 2004;42(1):15–8.

12. Feng S, He Q, Fan Y, et al. Nasal endoscopic findings and nasal symptoms in patients with asthma: a clinical study from a rhinological perspective. Allergol Immunopathol (Madr). 2015;43(1):42–7. https://doi.org/10.1016/j.aller.2013.10.005.

13. Chong LY, Head K, Hopkins C, et al. Different types of intranasal steroids for chronic rhinosinusitis (Review). Cochrane Database Syst Rev. 2016;4:CD011993. https://doi.org/10.1002/14651858.CD011993.pub2.www.cochranelibrary.com.

14. Chong LY, Head K, Hopkins C, Philpott C, Schilder AGM, Burton MJ. Intranasal steroids versus placebo or no intervention for chronic rhinosinusitis (Review) Cochrane Database Syst Rev. 2016;(4). https://doi.org/10.1002/14651858.CD011996.pub2.www.cochranelibrary.com.

15. Irvin CG, Mohapatra S, Peters SP. HHS public access. 2016;135(3):701–9. https://doi.org/10.1016/j.jaci.2014.06.038.Efficacy.

16. Lohia S, Schlosser RJ, Soler ZM. Impact of intranasal corticosteroids on asthma outcomes in allergic rhinitis: a meta-analysis. Allergy. 2013;68(5):569–79. https://doi.org/10.1111/all.12124.

17. Chong LY, Head K, Hopkins C, Philpott C, Burton MJ. Short-course oral steroids alone for chronic rhinosinusitis. Cochrane Database Syst Rev. 2015;2015(12). https://doi.org/10.1002/14651858.CD011991.

18. Hissaria P, Smith W, Wormald PJ, et al. Short course of systemic corticosteroids in sinonasal polyposis: a double-blind, randomized, placebo-controlled trial with evaluation of outcome measures. J Allergy Clin Immunol. 2006;118(1):128–33. https://doi.org/10.1016/j.jaci.2006.03.012.

19. Vaidyanathan S, Barnes M, Williamson P, Hopkinson P, Donnan PT, Lipworth B. Treatment of chronic rhinosinusitis with nasal polyposis with oral steroids followed by topical steroids: a randomized trial. Ann Intern Med. 2011;154(5):293–302. https://doi.org/10.7326/0003-4819-154-5-201103010-00003.

20. Ecevit MC, Erdag TK, Dogan E, Sutay S. Effect of steroids for nasal polyposis surgery: a placebo-controlled, randomized, double-blind study. Laryngoscope. 2015;125(9):2041–5. https://doi.org/10.1002/lary.25352.

21. Bülbül T, Bülbül ÖG, Güçlü O, Bilsel AS, Gürsan SÖ. Effect of glucocorticoids on nasal polyposis, with detection of inflammatory response by measurement of nitric oxide levels in nasal polyp tissue. J Laryngol Otol. 2013;127(6):584–9. https://doi.org/10.1017/S002221511300073X.

22. Rowe BH, Spooner CH, Ducharme FM, Bretzlaff JA, Bota GW. Corticosteroids for preventing relapse following acute exacerbations of asthma. Cochrane Database Syst Rev. 2007;(3). https://doi.org/10.1002/14651858.CD000195.pub2.

23. Normansell R, Kew KM, Mansour G. Different oral corticosteroid regimens for acute asthma. Cochrane Database Syst Rev. 2016;2016(5). https://doi.org/10.1002/14651858.CD011801.pub2.

24. Global strategy for asthma management and prevention. Glob Initiat Asthma. 2019. https://doi.org/10.1016/S0335-7457(96)80056-6.

25. Rudmik L, Soler ZM. Medical therapies for adult chronic sinusitis a systematic review. JAMA – J Am Med Assoc. 2015;314(9):926–39. https://doi.org/10.1001/jama.2015.7544.

26. Chauhan BF, Ducharme FM. Anti-leukotriene agents compared to inhaled corticosteroids in the management of recurrent and/or chronic asthma in adults and children. Cochrane Database Syst Rev. 2012;(5). https://doi.org/10.1002/14651858.CD002314.pub3.

27. Chauhan BF, Raja Ben Salah, Ducharme FM. Addition of anti-leukotriene agents to inhaled corticosteroids for adults and adolescents with persistent asthma. Cochrane Database Syst Rev. 2017;(3). https://doi.org/10.1002/14651858.CD010347.pub2.

28. Perez-Novo CA, Watelet JB, Claeys C, Van Cauwenberge P, Bachert C. Prostaglandin, leukotriene, and lipoxin balance in chronic rhinosinusitis with and without nasal polyposis. J Allergy Clin Immunol. 2005;115(6):1189–96. https://doi.org/10.1016/j.jaci.2005.02.029.

29. Chao S-S, Graham SM, Brown CL, Kline JN, Hussain I. Cysteinyl leukotriene 1 receptor expression in nasal polyps. Ann Otol Rhinol Laryngol. 2006;115(5):394–7. https://doi.org/10.1177/000348940611500513.

30. Wentzel JL, Soler ZM, DeYoung K, Nguyen SA, Lohia S, Schlosser RJ. Leukotriene antagonists in nasal polyposis: a meta-analysis and systematic review. Am J Rhinol Allergy. 2013;27(6):482–9. https://doi.org/10.2500/ajra.2013.27.3976.

31. Van ZT, Gevaert P, Holtappels G, et al. Oral steroids and doxycycline: two different approaches to treat nasal polyps. J Allergy Clin Immunol. 2010;125(5):1069–1076.e4. https://doi.org/10.1016/j.jaci.2010.02.020.

32. Head K, Chong LYL, Piromchai P, et al. Systemic and topical antibiotics for chronic rhinosinusitis (Review) summary of findings for the main comparison. Cochrane Database Syst Rev. 2016;2016(4). https://doi.org/10.1002/14651858.CD011994.pub2.www.cochranelibrary.com.

33. Haxel BR, Clemens M, Karaiskaki N, Dippold U, Kettern L, Mann WJ. Controlled trial for long-term low-dose erythromycin after sinus surgery for chronic rhinosinusitis. Laryngoscope. 2015;125(5):1048–55. https://doi.org/10.1002/lary.25052.

34. Varvyanskaya A, Lopatin A. Efficacy of long-term low-dose macrolide therapy in preventing early recurrence of nasal polyps after endoscopic sinus surgery. Int Forum Allergy Rhinol. 2014;4(7):533–41. https://doi.org/10.1002/alr.21318.

35. Barshak MB, Durand ML. The role of infection and antibiotics in chronic rhinosinusitis. Laryngoscope Investig Otolaryngol. 2017;2(1):36–42. https://doi.org/10.1002/lio2.61.

36. Kraft M, Cassell GH, Jane H, et al. Detection of mycoplasma pneumoniae in the airways of adults with chronic asthma. Am J Respir Crit Care Med. 1998;158(3):998–1001. https://doi.org/10.1164/ajrccm.158.3.9711092.

37. Sutherland ER, Martin RJ. Asthma and atypical bacterial infection. Chest. 2007;132(6):1962–6. https://doi.org/10.1378/chest.06-2415.

38. Kew KM, Undela K, Kotortsi I, Ferrara G. Macrolides for chronic asthma. Cochrane Database Syst Rev. 2015;2015(9). https://doi.org/10.1002/14651858.CD002997.pub4.
39. Nelson HS, Hamilos DL, Corsello PR, Levesque NV, Buchmeier AD, Bucher BL. A double-blind study of troleandomycin and methylprednisolone in asthmatic subjects who require daily corticosteroids. Am Rev Respir Dis. 1993;147(2):398–404. https://doi.org/10.1164/ajrccm/147.2.398.
40. Kamada AK, Hill MR, Iklé DN, Brenner AM, Szefler SJ. Efficacy and safety of low-dose troleandomycin therapy in children with severe, steroid-requiring asthma. J Allergy Clin Immunol. 1993;91(4):873–82. https://doi.org/10.1016/0091-6749(93)90345-G.
41. Wang X, Luo J, Wang D, Liu B, Liu C. The efficacy and safety of long-term add-on treatment of azithromycin in asthma. Medicine (Baltimore). 2019;98(38):e17190.
42. Zhang W, Lin C, Sampath V, Nadeau K. Impact of allergen immunotherapy in allergic asthma. Immunotherapy. 2018;10(7):579–93. https://doi.org/10.2217/imt-2017-0138.
43. Jutel M, Agache I, Bonini S, et al. International consensus on allergen immunotherapy II: mechanisms, standardization, and pharmacoeconomics. J Allergy Clin Immunol. 2016;137(2):358–68. https://doi.org/10.1016/j.jaci.2015.12.1300.
44. Wheatley LM, Togias A. Clinical practice. Allergic rhinitis. N Engl J Med. 2015;372(5):456–63. https://doi.org/10.1056/NEJMcp1412282.
45. Moller C, Dreborg S, Ferdousi HA, et al. Pollen immunotherapy reduces the development of asthma in children with seasonal rhinoconjunctivitis (the PAT-study). J Allergy Clin Immunol. 2002;109(2):251–6. https://doi.org/10.1067/mai.2002.121317.
46. Jacobsen L, Niggemann B, Dreborg S, et al. Specific immunotherapy has long-term preventive effect of seasonal and perennial asthma: 10-year follow-up on the PAT study. Allergy. 2007;62(8):943–8. https://doi.org/10.1111/j.1398-9995.2007.01451.x.
47. Zielen S, Devillier P, Heinrich J, Richter H, Wahn U. Sublingual immunotherapy provides long-term relief in allergic rhinitis and reduces the risk of asthma: a retrospective, real-world database analysis. Allergy. 2018;73(1):165–77. https://doi.org/10.1111/all.13213.
48. Virchow JC, Backer V, Kuna P, et al. Efficacy of a house dust mite sublingual allergen immunotherapy tablet in adults with allergic asthma: a randomized clinical trial. JAMA – J Am Med Assoc. 2016;315(16):1715–25. https://doi.org/10.1001/jama.2016.3964.
49. Fajt ML, Wenzel SE. Biologic therapy in asthma: entering the new age of personalized medicine. J Asthma. 2014;51(7):669–76. https://doi.org/10.3109/02770903.2014.910221.
50. Grundmann SA, Hemfort PB, Luger TA, Brehler R. Anti-IgE (omalizumab): a new therapeutic approach for chronic rhinosinusitis. J Allergy Clin Immunol. 2008;121(1):257–8. https://doi.org/10.1016/j.jaci.2007.09.036.
51. Smith KA, Pulsipher A, Gabrielsen DA, Alt JA. Biologics in chronic rhinosinusitis: an update and thoughts for future directions. Am J Rhinol Allergy. 2018;32(5):412–23. https://doi.org/10.1177/1945892418787132.
52. Gevaert P, Calus L, Van Zele T, et al. Omalizumab is effective in allergic and nonallergic patients with nasal polyps and asthma. J Allergy Clin Immunol. 2013;131(1):110–6.e1. https://doi.org/10.1016/j.jaci.2012.07.047.
53. Chandra RK, Clavenna M, Samuelson M, Tanner SB, Turner JH. Impact of omalizumab therapy on medication requirements for chronic rhinosinusitis. Int Forum Allergy Rhinol. 2016;6(5):472–7. https://doi.org/10.1002/alr.21685.
54. Gevaert P, Van Bruaene N, Cattaert T, et al. Mepolizumab, a humanized anti-IL-5 mAb, as a treatment option for severe nasal polyposis. J Allergy Clin Immunol. 2011;128(5):988–9. https://doi.org/10.1016/j.jaci.2011.07.056.
55. Laviolette M, Gossage DL, Gauvreau G, et al. Effects of benralizumab on airway eosinophils in asthmatic patients with sputum eosinophilia. J Allergy Clin Immunol. 2013;132(5):1086–1096.e5. https://doi.org/10.1016/j.jaci.2013.05.020.
56. Bachert C, Mannent L, Naclerio RM, et al. Effect of subcutaneous dupilumab on nasal polyp burden in patients with chronic sinusitis and nasal polyposis: a randomized clinical trial. JAMA. 2016;315(5):469–79. https://doi.org/10.1001/jama.2015.19330.
57. Chiu AG, Palmer JN, Woodworth BA, et al. Baby shampoo nasal irrigations for the symptomatic post-functional endoscopic sinus surgery patient. Am J Rhinol. 2008;22(1):34–7. https://doi.org/10.2500/ajr.2008.22.3122.

Chapter 6

Asthma and Chronic Rhinosinusitis: Surgical Management and Outcomes

Kevin Li, Viraj Patel, and Waleed M. Abuzeid

Key Concepts
- Endoscopic sinus surgery (ESS) is often indicated in patients whose CRS fails to improve with appropriate medical therapy.
- ESS improves CRS outcome measures while also reducing asthma symptoms and dependence on asthma medications.
- Extended endoscopic procedures, including Draf 2b and Draf 3 frontal sinus surgery, can significantly improve sinonasal outcomes.

Surgical Approach

Timing of Surgery

In the context of the unified airway theory, it has been found that asthma and other upper airway conditions such as chronic rhinosinusitis (CRS) are related. Among patients with asthma, the prevalence of CRS is estimated to be approximately 22%–45%—with a higher prevalence in patients with more severe asthma [1,

K. Li · V. Patel
Department of Otorhinolaryngology: Head and Neck Surgery, Division of Rhinology and Skull Base Surgery, Montefiore Medical Center, Albert Einstein College of Medicine, Bronx, NY, USA

W. M. Abuzeid (✉)
Division of Rhinology and Skull Base Surgery, Department of Otolaryngology: Head and Neck Surgery, University of Washington, Seattle, WA, USA
e-mail: wabuzeid@uw.edu

© Springer Nature Switzerland AG 2020
D. A. Gudis, R. J. Schlosser (eds.), *The Unified Airway*,
https://doi.org/10.1007/978-3-030-50330-7_6

2]—compared to the prevalence of CRS in the general population, which is estimated to be 10%–12% [3]. Patients with both asthma and chronic rhinosinusitis generally have worse asthma symptoms and overall worse quality of life (QOL) [4]. Furthermore, having CRS with nasal polyposis (CRSwNP) is associated with more severe sinus symptoms and more severe asthma [5]. Aspirin-exacerbated respiratory disease (AERD) was also found to be twice as prevalent in patients with severe asthma compared to patients with less severe asthma variants and was diagnosed in approximately 10% of patients with CRSwNP [6]. Clinically, CRSwNP trends toward worse preoperative QOL scores when compared with CRS without nasal polyposis (CRSsNP) [7]. Patients with CRSwNP also have greater improvements in QOL measurements after surgical intervention compared to patients with CRSsNP [7, 8].

The current treatment paradigm for CRSwNP or CRSsNP with or without associated asthma or AERD is to treat initially with medical therapy, which is discussed in a separate chapter. However, if medical therapy fails, endoscopic sinus surgery (ESS) can be offered as an option. Because surgery does not correct the underlying inflammatory component of CRS, it serves as an adjunct to medical treatment rather than a replacement. There are no standard criteria for which patients are offered surgery or for the appropriate timing for surgical intervention. Furthermore, the lack of comprehensive guidelines contributes to the large geographic variation in surgical rates and in quality of care [9]. The decision to proceed with surgical intervention is multifactorial and depends on a variety of patient factors including sense of risk, cultural factors, cost of treatment, and patient interest [10].

In a prospective, multicenter, observational cohort study by Schlosser et al., it was found that patients with asthma and CRS experienced significant improvement in asthma symptoms, sinus symptoms, and QOL after ESS as measured by the Asthma Control Test (ACT), Sinonasal Outcome Test (SNOT-22), and Mini Asthma QOL Questionnaire scores. Patients with uncontrolled asthma at baseline received the most benefit after ESS [11]. In a prior study by Chen et al. examining ACT outcomes after ESS, there was no significant improvement in postoperative ACT scores [12]. However, in their study cohort, only 11% of patients had uncontrolled asthma as opposed to 51% in the study by Schlosser et al. Overall, these studies suggest not only that patients with uncontrolled asthma are more likely to benefit from ESS but also that this group of patients may benefit from earlier surgery. Earlier surgery also benefits patients with uncontrolled asthma who are dependent on corticosteroid therapy as there is evidence that ESS reduces steroid dependency [11].

Hopkins et al. evaluated the impact time-to-ESS had on the outcomes of CRS by comparing patients who underwent surgery within a year of the diagnosis (early cohort) with those who had surgery at least 5 years after diagnosis (late cohort) retrospectively as well as prospectively using SNOT-22 scores [13, 14]. In the early cohort, fewer patients returned for CRS-related care in the 5-year postoperative period and, overall, these patients had significantly fewer number of hospital visits and prescriptions [13]. In a sub-analysis of patients in the early and late cohort with or without asthma, patients with asthma in the late cohort had the highest postoperative needs and highest preoperative SNOT-22 scores of all groups. It was also found that there were significantly more patients with asthma in the late cohort. Although it has been shown that patients with higher preoperative SNOT-22 scores tend to have more significant postoperative improvement, in this study, the late cohort—which had the higher preoperative SNOT-22—improved postoperatively, but not as significantly as the early cohort [9, 10, 15, 16]. These findings together suggest that delays in performing ESS for CRS, particularly in patients with asthma, may reduce the extent of symptomatic benefit from surgery and may also significantly reduce the percentage of patients who experience sustained clinical improvement [14]. Smith et al. conducted a prospective non-randomized multi-institutional study that provides additional evidence that earlier surgery, after failing appropriate medical therapy, is beneficial over continued medical therapy [17, 18].

Although there is substantial evidence that shows the integral role ESS plays in optimizing the QOL of patients with AERD, it is important to understand that these patients often have more severe disease preoperatively and may have less significant improvement postoperatively compared to patients without AERD. Patients with AERD often suffer from poor symptom control on medical therapy alone and have a higher propensity for failing initial ESS. Therefore, a push for earlier and more extensive surgery may be more appropriate to improve their QOL [19]. It has been shown that AERD patients have less significant improvement after ESS compared to those with asthma who are aspirin tolerant, which may suggest this group requires a more aggressive approach [20]. A further benefit of ESS in AERD relates to the efficacy of aspirin desensitization. Shah et al. found that ESS performed within weeks of aspirin desensitization significantly improves patient tolerance of aspirin desensitization and can effectively convert those who failed aspirin desensitization prior to surgery to a more responsive phenotype [21]. This finding argues not only for the use of ESS in the management of AERD but also for earlier surgical intervention as a means of enhancing postoperative medical management. Overall, patients with AERD may benefit from early and aggressive surgical therapy.

Indications for Routine Surgery

ESS is targeted toward optimizing the ventilation and drainage of the paranasal sinuses through the widening of the sinus ostia and removal of inflamed bone and soft tissue components. Surgery also enhances the delivery of topical corticosteroids into the paranasal sinuses, thereby improving control of the inflammation at the level of the sinus epithelium [22–24]. The extent of surgery is often tailored to the extent of sinus disease as determined by nasal endoscopy and CT findings [25]. For the purposes of this chapter, routine ESS is defined as bilateral maxillary antrostomy, total ethmoidectomy, sphenoidotomy, and/or frontal sinusotomy but does not include extended sinus procedures such as Draf IIb, Draf III, maxillary mega-antrostomy, or medial maxillectomy.

The indications for routine ESS in asthmatic patients with CRS or in those with AERD are similar to the indications for surgery in the CRS population. Prior work has cited failure of maximal medical therapy as an indication for ESS. Given the literature cited above, there is no consensus on what maximal medical therapy entails, and surgeons should aim to avoid protracted trials of maximal medical therapy. In an effort to introduce terminology that would minimize unnecessary delay in surgical treatment, a recent international consensus statement introduced the term appropriate medical therapy (AMT) [26]. This attempts to balance the appropriate use of conservative medical modalities prior to ESS with suboptimal delays in surgical management that may adversely impact patient outcomes. A trial of AMT should, generally, include a 3–4-week trial of intranasal corticosteroids, saline irrigations, a single course of oral corticosteroids, and an optional trial of oral antibiotics for patients with CRSwNP, which includes the AERD cohort. For those with CRSsNP and asthma, AMT entails intranasal corticosteroids, saline irrigations, and oral antibiotics—either a short course of a broad-spectrum systemic antibiotic or a ≥3-week course of a low-dose anti-inflammatory antibiotic such as clarithromycin—with the optional use of oral corticosteroids [9, 26]. Patients who fail the trial of AMT are deemed candidates for routine ESS.

Efforts have been made to define treatment failure in a more objective fashion. Rudmik et al. published a landmark paper using the RAND/UCLA appropriateness methodology to define criteria for ESS [9]. By analyzing 624 clinical scenarios evenly split between CRSwNP and CRSsNP coupled with a Delphi ranking process involving an international panel of 10 experts in CRS, the investigators concluded that ESS should be offered to adults patients with CRS when the Lund-Mackay CT score is ≥1 and a post-AMT total SNOT-22 score ≥20 with the course of AMT tailored to the presence or absence of polyps as above. There are scenarios in which proceeding with ESS, without a preceding trial of AMT, is appropriate. In the context of CRS and asthma or AERD, the presence of mucocele, concurrent allergic fungal rhinosinusitis, or other complications related to the extension of disease beyond the sinuses, proceeding with ESS, is indicated [27].

In patients with CRSwNP and asthma, both those with and without aspirin intolerance improved after routine ESS, suggesting that routine surgery can be appropriate for patients with CRSwNP and concurrent asthma as well as those with AERD [28]. In the AERD population, failure of aspirin treatment or ongoing severe underlying aspirin sensitivity may be an indication for surgery. Given that aspirin therapy is critical to the maintenance of disease control in AERD, converting patients to an aspirin-tolerant phenotype so that they can tolerate aspirin maintenance therapy is a management goal [29]. To this end, ESS is indicated in patients unable to tolerate initiation of aspirin therapy as surgery can convert patients who previously failed aspirin desensitization to a more tolerant phenotype who can take aspirin maintenance therapy [21, 30]. Typically, these aspirin treatment "failures" will have markedly elevated levels of baseline serum IgE which, if validated in additional studies, may prove to be an objective marker for proceeding with ESS in AERD cases.

Indications for Extended Surgery

The success rate of ESS in controlling CRS symptoms that are refractory to medical therapy approaches 80% [31]. Therefore, a significant proportion of patients fail ESS and may benefit from extended ESS [32]. Indeed, patients with a high inflammatory load, which typically involves high-grade eosinophilic inflammation as is seen in AERD, tend to fail because routine ESS may incompletely address the inflamed mucosa and may benefit from a more aggressive surgical approach [33]. Patients with refractory CRS who have failed both medical therapy and routine ESS with appropriate postoperative maintenance therapy should be considered for extended ESS.

CRS with asthma predisposes to recalcitrant CRS with more severe symptoms, higher incidence of recurrence, and higher rates of revision surgery [29, 34–38]. Among these patients, those with AERD have worse sinonasal disease compared to aspirin-tolerant asthma patients and, furthermore, do not respond as well to routine ESS [28, 29, 39]. AERD patients undergoing ESS have an approximate 90% polyp recurrence rate within 5 years and markedly higher rates of revision ESS [35]. This patient population may benefit from more extended ESS, though the timing of such surgery remains a subject of study. At present, extended surgery is typically considered in a revision scenario following the failure of medical therapy and routine ESS though there is an ongoing study evaluating the utility of extended ESS as a first-line surgical treatment in AERD.

Extended maxillary sinus surgery includes endoscopic maxillary mega-antrostomy, modified medial maxillectomy, and inferior meatal antrostomy. These extended procedures help facilitate gravity-dependent drainage and enhance access for nasal irrigations and topical medication delivery. In some patients, particularly in situations where the diseased mucosa is removed, there is volume reduction of the maxillary sinuses through osteoneogenesis, which can reduce mucus accumulation and bacterial colonization [40]. Friedman and Katsantonis evaluated patients with recalcitrant maxillary sinusitis who failed to improve after undergoing maxillary antrostomy and found that the rate of polyp recurrence was significantly decreased after marsupializing the maxillary sinus to the posterior nasal vault and removing all residual diseased mucosa including polyps, mucoceles, and hyperplastic epithelium [41]. Cho et al. evaluated 28 patients with recalcitrant maxillary sinusitis who failed routine maxillary antrostomy and found that endoscopic maxillary mega-antrostomy (EMMA) was both safe and efficacious. Approximately 75% of patients reported complete resolution of symptoms, 25% reported partial improvement, and 0% reported worse symptoms [42]. In a follow-up study by the same group, EMMA continued to show efficacy in the original study cohort and in an expanded population with long-term maintenance of symptom improvement as measured by SNOT-22 and sustained improvement in objective endoscopic and CT scores [43].

First described in 1995, radical ethmoidectomy, also termed nasalization, involves a total ethmoidectomy followed by mucosal stripping, with or without middle turbinate resection. This technique is indicated for recalcitrant ethmoid polyposis as occurs in the setting of AERD and severe CRSwNP [44]. Compared to standard total ethmoidectomy, nasal polyp recurrence rates were significantly lower after nasalization with enhanced resolution of polyp-related hyposmia and objective improvement in validated endoscopic and CT scores [45, 46]. In the hands of a skilled sinus surgeon, nasalization was found to be as safe as routine total ethmoidectomy [45].

Chronic recalcitrant sphenoid sinusitis is a feature of recalcitrant CRS with asthma and AERD. There is a paucity of literature evaluating the efficacy of extended sphenoidotomy techniques. These extended sphenoidotomy techniques typically involve the so-called sphenoid drill-out as an interval step between standard sphenoidotomy and sphenoid nasalization. In the drill-out procedure, the bilateral sphenoid ostium is enlarged by removing the sphenoid face superiorly to the planum, inferiorly to the sinus floor, and laterally to the sphenoid lateral walls with the removal of the intersinus septum and performance of a posterior septectomy [47]. Sphenoid nasalization is the corollary to Draf III frontal sinusotomy and involves performing the aforementioned drill-out with the removal of the sphenoid sinus floor so as to marsupialize a common sphenoid cavity [48]. The outcomes of these procedures have yet to be comprehensively evaluated.

Benefits of Draf 2b and Draf III in CRSwNP

The frontal sinus is the most likely sinus to demonstrate loss of disease control after standard (Draf 2a) frontal sinusotomy with obstructive polyposis and stenosis particularly common in severe CRSwNP and AERD [35, 49]. In AERD patients, the polyp recurrence rate over 5 years was 90% after ESS with a surgical revision rate of 89% [35]. Nasal polyps, AERD, and asthma have all been associated with failure of primary frontal sinusotomy [50]. Furthermore, failure of an initial frontal sinusotomy is an independent risk factor for failure of a revision Draf 2a [51]. Consequently, more extensive frontal sinus surgery is often indicated in CRSwNP and AERD patients who fail an initial Draf 2a frontal sinusotomy [52].

The options for extended frontal sinusotomy include Draf 2b or Draf III (endoscopic modified Lothrop procedure; EMLP) techniques. In a retrospective cohort study comparing Draf 2b sinusotomy to EMLP in 38 CRS patients undergoing revision ESS—including approximately 20% of patients in each treatment arm with asthma and about 20% with AERD—followed over a mean of 15.6 months, both techniques were associated with significant symptomatic improvement [53]. The Draf 2b cohort had a greater improvement than EMLP patients within 1–3 months of surgery attributed to the reduced mucosal removal and potentially faster healing in the former group. The magnitude of symptom improvement equalized at later time points, and there was no significant difference between Draf 2b and EMLP in patency or revision rates leading the authors to suggest the Draf 2b as a less aggressive alternative to the EMLP for recalcitrant CRS [53].

To date, the evidence supporting the use of the Draf 2b in lieu of EMLP is limited. In contrast, there is abundant data demonstrating the benefits of EMLP in the management of patients with recalcitrant CRS. The EMLP facilitates the removal of inflammatory mediators in sinonasal mucosa, reducing the "inflammatory load" resulting from the proinflammatory tissue environment created by eosinophils and—more so than the Draf 2b—allowing for the removal of osteitic bone and polyps that may also contribute to inflammation and anatomic obstruction of the frontal recess [33]. Furthermore, EMLP enhances postoperative debridement and access for topical irrigation to the frontal sinuses [24]. A recent meta-analysis on EMLP incorporated a subgroup analysis of 7 studies consisting of 357 patients all of whom had CRS [52]. Among these patients, 53.8% had asthma, and 17.4% had AERD. Symptom improvement was 75.9% over a mean follow-up of 31.5 months. The polyp recurrence rate was 23.1%, which compares favorably to the 40% recurrence rate in CRS patients followed over 18 months after ESS, particularly considering that this rate was achieved with a relatively high burden of AERD in the study population [52, 54].

AERD has been independently associated with symptom improvement after EMLP potentially related to the worse symptoms seen in these patients preoperatively relative to non-AERD cases and the greater opportunity for symptom improvement post-ESS [52, 55]. This symptom improvement was noted to be superior in asthma or aspirin-sensitive patients undergoing EMLP compared to AERD patients treated with routine revision ESS [56].

The resilience of EMLP for CRS is well established. Long-term stenosis occurs in 17.1% of cases and complete closure in 3.9%. Consequently, the revision ESS rate after performing an EMLP is only 9.0% [52]. AERD has previously been associated with an increased risk of surgical failure after EMLP [57]. However, this is not a consistent finding with several studies indicating that neither asthma or aspirin sensitivity was associated with stenosis or closure of the EMLP [52, 58–60]. Furthermore, recent evidence suggests that the presence of asthma or aspirin sensitivity is not necessarily associated with revision of EMLP potentially due to changing trends in surgery with surgeons creating maximal openings of the neo-ostium in the setting of AERD and modifying their techniques to use mucosal grafts, further reducing the risk of ostial stenosis [52, 61]. The primary disadvantage of the EMLP in appropriately selected patients is the significant 2.5% risk of CSF leak when the procedure is performed for CRS, limiting the use of this technique to experienced surgeons [52].

Overall, there is considerable evidence supporting the use of the EMLP and, to a lesser extent, Draf 2b in the management of CRS with concurrent asthma and AERD.

Postoperative Maintenance Therapy

Postoperative maintenance therapy is an essential component in the treatment of CRS and AERD for the prevention of disease recurrence. After ESS, the underlying inflammatory processes of CRS remain, and continued medical therapy is crucial [62–64]. While there is an abundance of literature guiding optimal postoperative maintenance therapy for CRS, with and without asthma, there is still a paucity of studies evaluating postoperative regimens in patients with AERD.

Nasal saline administration is a key component of postoperative maintenance therapy in patients after ESS. Typically, nasal saline is administered via high-volume irrigation achieved through the use of a squeeze bottle or similar device [65,

66]. These nasal irrigations have the added advantage of optimizing the delivery of topical medications throughout the sinonasal cavities during the postoperative period and beyond [67]. Generally, the mechanism of action of nasal irrigation is through the liquefaction of nasal secretions, direct clearance of mucus and antigens, removal of bacterial biofilms and inflammatory mediators, and concomitant improvement in mucociliary clearance [68, 69]. This may be synergistic with the baseline improvement in mucociliary clearance observed in patients with CRS treated with ESS [70]. Moreover, it is thought that there is a vasoconstrictive effect of saline irrigation that acts to decongest the sinonasal cavity [68].

Squeeze bottles or neti pots have proven superior to other delivery systems, including nebulizers and pressurized sprays, in delivering saline and medications to the paranasal sinuses [71, 72]. In one randomized controlled trial (RCT), high-volume, low-pressure nasal irrigation was more effective than saline sprays for CRS as measured by a mean improvement in SNOT-20 scores of 12.2–16.2 points measured at multiple time points over an 8-week follow-up period [73]. Patients randomized to saline irrigations, interestingly, did not change the amount of adjuvant topical medication use compared to patients randomized to saline spray. However, the authors note that this finding could be a result of a broader inclusion criteria and an underpowered study for the detection of this specific outcome [73]. In another single-blind RCT, high-volume low-pressure saline irrigation delivered by squeeze bottle was superior to nasal saline sprays for up to 12 weeks postoperatively with significantly better modified Lund-Kennedy endoscopic scores in the early postoperative period [74].

The observed superiority in symptom scores and endoscopic appearance observed with high-volume sinus irrigation may be related to enhanced sinus penetration. A cadaveric study compared penetration of radiopaque contrast delivered via pressurized spray versus neti pot versus squeeze bottle after ESS and found significant differences in distribution, with neti pot superior to squeeze bottle which was, in turn, significantly better than pressurized spray [71]. The superiority of high-volume irrigations in penetrating the frontal sinus has also been demonstrated in similar cadaveric work [75, 76]. Interestingly, head position also appears to play a role in the penetration of saline irrigation, with optimal positioning for the frontal sinuses thought to be 90° to the vertical axis [77].

Cadaveric studies are limited in that they only reveal the final location of dyes and not the dynamics of the irrigation. Recent advances in computational fluid dynamics (CFD) have led to the creation of sinonasal irrigation flow simulation models with adjustable parameters [22, 78]. In a CFD study where all the paranasal sinuses were surgically opened in a cadaver, Craig et al. found that post-sphenoidotomy, nose-to-ceiling head position allowed complete nasal irrigation into the sphenoid sinuses, likely due to its gravity-dependent position. In contrast, a nose-to-floor position resulted in zero penetration into the sphenoid sinuses. The other sinuses did not differ significantly in irrigation penetration between head positions [79]. Zhao et al. found that a Draf III frontal sinusotomy drastically improved irrigation to the frontal sinuses in a CFD study, which corroborates a previous study by Harvey et al. [71, 78]. This finding is particularly important in the context of

CRSwNP and concurrent asthma or AERD where extended frontal sinus surgery may be both indicated and performed at an earlier stage than in other less severe forms of CRS. Surprisingly, Zhao et al. also found that the removal of the superior and intersinus septums resulted in less irrigation of the maxillary sinus due to premature spillage across the septum and reduced irrigation to the more posteriorly located sinuses. The authors believe that less aggressive surgery, such as Draf II procedures, may avoid this issue [78]. In practicality, the extent of sinus surgery continues to be a debated topic as it may be that enhancing delivery to one sinus could compromise irrigant delivery to other sinuses. Furthermore, the results of CFD studies have occasionally differed from prior cadaveric and in vivo studies highlighting the need for the development of more representative experimental models. Nevertheless, taken together, the data indicates that the efficacy of nasal irrigation depends on the specific sinus being targeted, irrigation volume, and irrigation pressure. Generally, nasal irrigation coupled with ESS provides better sinus penetration irrespective of head position [24, 80, 81].

Topical corticosteroids are also critical to the control of mucosal inflammation post-ESS. Corticosteroids are routinely delivered by nasal irrigation or as an aerosolized spray after ESS and are beneficial in reducing polyp burden and recurrence rates [82–84]. Multiple studies have shown that postoperative steroid irrigation improves symptom scores such as SNOT-22, endoscopy scores, and prognosis. ESS also improves the effectiveness of steroid irrigations, likely due to improved access as discussed above [85–87]. Overall, the data suggests that corticosteroid irrigations are superior to corticosteroid sprays. Harvey et al., in a double-blinded RCT of patients post-ESS with CRS—with and without asthma—showed that high-volume (240 mL) mometasone nasal rinses compared to mometasone sprays statistically improved nasal obstruction, measured on a visual analogue scale (VAS) (-69.91 ± 29.37), Lund-Mackay scores (-12.07 ± 4.43), and modified Lund-Kennedy scores (7.33 ± 11.55). The investigators note that this may be secondary to inadequate penetration of aerosolized corticosteroid into the paranasal sinuses despite the higher concentration of corticosteroid in sprays relative to irrigation [88, 89]. Neubauer et al., in another RCT of post-ESS patients diagnosed with CRSwNP, with and without asthma or AERD, demonstrated that patients who were treated with budesonide delivered via a mucosal atomization device had greater improvement of SNOT-22 and Lund-Kennedy scores compared to fluticasone sprays [90]. Though this study further reinforces the conclusion that corticosteroid nasal sprays are an inferior method of delivering corticosteroids to the paranasal sinuses, the absence of a budesonide irrigation arm limits the ability to define the most advantageous delivery method.

From a tolerability and safety standpoint, the risk of mild epistaxis with topical corticosteroid sprays has been well established. Furthermore, corticosteroid sprays have little effect on the hypothalamic-pituitary-adrenal axis (HPAA) or on intraocular pressure [91, 92]. Given the increased use of corticosteroid irrigations over sprays post-ESS due to the aforementioned advantages, investigators have attempted to define the safety profile of these rinses. In one retrospective analysis, 23% of patients were found to have abnormally low stimulated cortisol levels without concomitant symptoms of adrenal suppression. Continued monitoring of this cohort did not reveal the development of frank clinical manifestations of adrenal insufficiency with continued use of the budesonide rinses [93]. The authors do note that concurrent use of nasal steroid sprays or pulmonary steroid inhalers with budesonide rinses was significantly associated with HPAA suppression, and other sources of exogenous steroid should always be considered in the management of post-ESS patients. The likelihood of systemic manifestations of corticosteroid irrigation use is unlikely given findings of a recent meta-analysis by Yoon et al. and an RCT by Huang et al. that found no risk of systemic steroid absorption with nasal irrigation over a mean follow-up time of 22 months [86, 94]. There is no evidence to date implicating corticosteroid nasal irrigations in elevations of intraocular pressure [93].

Overall, the literature supports the use of corticosteroid irrigations or, potentially, atomized corticosteroid in the postoperative management of CRS patients, including those with asthma or AERD, as a superior adjunct when compared to corticosteroid sprays.

Benefits of Endoscopic Sinus Surgery in CRS with Asthma and AERD

ESS has demonstrated improvements in QOL metrics including SNOT-22, Rhinosinusitis Disability Index (RSDI), and Chronic Sinusitis Survey scores and is associated with sustained improvements in objective measures of disease severity including Lund-Kennedy nasal endoscopy scores and Lund-Mackay CT scores in patients with CRS and concurrent asthma and in those with AERD [18, 36, 95, 96]. Smith et al. ran a prospective, multi-institutional study with 1-year follow-up of CRS patients, with or without asthma, that failed medical management to compare continued medical therapy versus ESS. The authors found that, at 1-year follow-up, patients who underwent ESS had much higher QOL measures compared to medically managed patients (total RSDI 22.3 ± 24.3 vs. 12.1 ± 19.5, respectively). This extended into a small cohort of patients who crossed over from medical management to surgical management, where QOL measures were stagnant on medical therapy and improved significantly when patients switched to surgical management (total RSDI 12.1 ± 19.5 vs. 20.6 ± 28.6, respectively) [18]. Critically, 17%–25% of patients undergoing ESS for CRS fail to have an improvement in QOL metrics [97, 98]. This highlights the need for improved stratification of surgical candidates into those most likely to demonstrate an improvement after ESS.

In patients with AERD, ESS allows a direct decrease in disease burden, reportedly reducing asthma symptoms by approximately 90%, and facilitates more effective medical treatment. Many studies have also noted the adjunctive benefit of aspirin desensitization after ESS. There is evidence that in patients with AERD, more aggressive extended endoscopic sinus surgery that widely opens all the sinuses reduces the rate of revision surgery and decreases the rate of polyp recurrence compared to standard sinus surgery [29, 57, 99]. Morrissey et al. attributed the difference in revision rates and polyp recurrence to the use of EMLP for frontal sinus disease [57]. This corroborates the meta-analysis by Abuzeid et al. that found EMLP efficacious for recalcitrant frontal sinus disease after failed primary ESS. Interestingly, aspirin sensitivity and asthma were both found to be significantly associated with post-EMLP symptom improvement [52]. In contrast, there is evidence that though ethmoidectomy can effectively treat frontal sinus disease in many cases of CRS, the presence of asthma, polyposis, or AERD curtails the benefit of limited ESS and patients with these characteristics will likely require direct addressal of the frontal sinus [100].

The effect of ESS on symptom-specific outcomes has been evaluated across multiple studies and reported in a systematic review [101]. Chester et al. evaluated 21 studies comprising 2070 patients with CRS with a mean follow-up time of 13.9 months after ESS and found all cardinal symptoms improved relative to preoperative baseline severity. Nasal obstruction improved the most followed by facial pain and postnasal discharge, while hyposmia and headache improved the least. Similarly, Amar et al. conducted a retrospective analysis examining outcomes of ESS on 22 AERD patients compared to CRS patients. One month following initial ESS, both groups had significant improvement in symptoms, but AERD patients had a higher prevalence of all cardinal symptoms except for postnasal discharge. Notably, anosmia was present in approximately 89% of postoperative AERD patients compared to 50% in non-AERD patients [39]. Though there is consistency in reported improvements in nasal obstruction, facial pressure, and nasal drainage after ESS, improvements in olfaction are less consistently reported. To illustrate, DeConde et al. found that ESS in a diverse population of patients with CRS— including those with or without asthma and patients with AERD--induced a three to four times higher likelihood of complete resolution in three of the four cardinal symptoms of disease. This improvement was significant when compared to symptoms in patients electing to continue medical therapy rather than undergo ESS. Specifically, there were improvements in nasal blockage, facial pain/pressure, and thick nasal discharge, but olfaction did not improve significantly [102].

ESS can be an effective treatment for hyposmia related to CRS and AERD [95, 103–108]. The literature suggests that there is improvement in olfaction within weeks of ESS that is sustained, in the majority of patients, for months to years [104, 109]. This appears to be true for varying CRS endotypes including eosinophilic, Th2-driven CRS and can be achieved through a variety of surgical techniques including procedures such as the "outside in" EMLP which is performed in close proximity to the olfactory fibers of the cribriform [105, 110]. However, based on a multi-institutional prospectively accrued cohort of CRS patients, only 38.6% with impaired olfaction returned to normal olfaction after ESS, and interestingly, this proportion was similar to the proportion of patients with normalization of olfaction undergoing medical therapy alone [102].

Among AERD patients, olfactory gains from ESS were found to be less than in those patients without AERD, as measured by odor discrimination, odor identification, odor threshold, and composite threshold-discrimination-identification (TDI) scores [111]. Patients with AERD had lower TDI scores postoperatively than those without AERD (12.81 ± 6.47 vs. 20.41 ± 6.97, respectively). Furthermore, compared to patients without AERD, olfactory function did not continue to change between the 3rd and 6th postoperative month. However, a meta-analysis of 31 studies by Kohli et al. found that both subjective and objective measures of olfaction improved after ESS and were, in fact, a clinically significant improvement. This analysis looked at SNOT-22 and VAS for subjective scores and Smell Identification Test and B-SIT for objective scoring. Moreover, the authors found that hyposmic patients and patients with nasal polyps had greater absolute improvements in their olfaction postoperatively [112]. Overall, the heterogeneity in olfactory outcomes may be related to heterogeneity in the study populations, with AERD patients seeming to fare worse after ESS and those with non-AERD polyposis doing better, as well as the underlying shortcomings of existing treatments in reversing irreversible damage to olfactory nerves in the presence of chronic inflammation [113].

Schlosser et al., in a systematic review, noted that depression is a comorbidity associated with CRS in 40% of cases [114]. Many of the symptoms of CRS or AERD, including olfactory loss, sleep disturbances, and concomitant asthma, may lead to higher depression scores and subsequently worse QOL [107, 111, 115–118]. Some of these contributing factors can be improved through ESS. For example, Alt et al. noted that ESS improved sleep quality as measured by the Pittsburgh Sleep Quality Index, but the presence of comorbid asthma was found to partially contribute to residual sleep dysfunction after ESS [118]. Though ESS appears to improve contributing factors, the evidence for definitive improvements in depression itself is more controversial. DeConde et al. did not report a difference in symptoms of depression between CRS patients treated with ESS or those treated with medical management [102]. Gudziol et al. found no significant difference in the Beck Depression Inventory score between patients with AERD and those that are aspirin tolerant [107]. Similarly, Adams et al. found that patients with CRS, though experiencing post-FESS improvements in objective measures of disease such as Lund-Kennedy score and RSDI, did not see a significant improvement in depression or anxiety when compared to nonsurgical patients [119]. Moreover, the improvement in quality-of-life scores, such as SNOT-22, was lower in patients with comorbid depression postoperatively than those without depression [120]. In contrast, Schlosser et al. found that surgical therapy for CRS increased Patient Health Questionnaire-2 scores—a measure of depressed mood and anhedonia—by approximately 50% [117]. In their systematic review, Schlosser et al. found patients treated with ESS with comorbid depression both started and ended treatment with worse CRS-specific QOL outcomes, but interestingly, the absolute level of improvement is similar between patients with or without comorbid depression [114]. In light of these contrasting findings, the association between surgical intervention for CRS and depression continues to be a focus of investigation.

In addition to the symptom-related impact of ESS, there is also an associated total economic burden that has been estimated to be tens of millions of US dollars

(USD) annually [121, 122]. In a 2015 systematic review of 44 articles, Smith et al. estimated that in 2014, the total annual medication cost for CRS was $22 million USD and that the average cost of a single ESS procedure in the United States was $8000 USD, which is multiple times the cost in other countries such as Canada. In comparison, prior to ESS, annual medication costs were estimated between $1500 and $2700 per patient per year, with a universal reduction of annual cost post-ESS [122]. Scangas et al. looked specifically at the cost-effectiveness of surgical intervention for CRSwNP patients with asthma. The authors found that ESS is cost-effective for patients with CRS, with or without asthma, compared to medical therapy. The comorbidity of asthma resulted in a higher burden for ESS of $12,066 per quality-adjusted life year (QALY) compared to $7369 per QALY for medical therapy, as measured by an incremental cost-effectiveness ratio. This is similar to their overall finding that ESS is cost-effective compared to medical therapy when they evaluated patients with CRS alone [123, 124]. Given the comorbidity rates with depression, Rudmik et al. evaluated associated productivity costs—noting that these can exceed direct medical costs—and found that patients with refractory CRS who underwent ESS reduced their mean annual productivity cost from $9190 to $3373 USD. This difference equates to approximately a $1.5 billion USD benefit to society per year when all the ESS procedures performed in the United States are considered. The authors point out that this finding reinforces the paradigm of attempting maximal medical therapy before ESS, but since ESS is more effective for refractory CRS, it is ultimately more cost-effective [125, 126].

The literature has shown ESS to be an extremely valuable therapy in patients with CRS and asthma or AERD. Not only does ESS improve both subjective and objective QOL measures, but also it directly reduces the burden of disease and improves the cardinal symptoms of CRS. The superiority of ESS and extended ESS in treating recalcitrant CRS with asthma or AERD over continued medical therapy is especially important when comorbid depression and the total economic burden of disease are considered.

Impact of Rhinologic Interventions on Medical Comorbidities

Asthma

Many studies have evaluated the impact of ESS on asthma. In patients with CRS and asthma, ESS produces a more significant improvement in asthma symptom scores than medical therapy for CRS [127–129]. A prospective analysis of 20 patients with CRS and asthma found that 85% of patients self-reported improvement in their asthma symptoms after ESS [130]. A larger cohort of 50 asthmatic patients with CRS demonstrated that ESS produced a 40% improvement in asthma control [131]. A multi-institutional prospective study showed that in CRS patients with uncontrolled asthma at baseline (ACT score <20), ESS produced a minimal clinically important difference 57% of the time on miniAQLQ testing and 50% of the time in ACT scores, suggesting that about half of patients with uncontrolled asthma see an improvement after ESS [11]. Senior et al. demonstrated that these symptom improvements in asthma control were sustained over a mean 6.5-year follow-up time after ESS [132]. Interestingly, patients who demonstrate a greater improvement in sinus symptom scores post-ESS tended to have a better improvement in their asthma symptoms, consistent with the unified airway theory and the anticipated reduction in pulmonary inflammation with enhanced control of sinonasal disease [133].

Studies have also shown that, in general, objective measures of asthma control such as peak expiratory flow remain improved for at least 1 year after ESS [127–129]. Some studies have also found objective, though not statistically significant, improvements in FEV1 values postoperatively [20, 134]. Interestingly, Chen et al. in their prospective non-randomized cohort of 27 CRS patients with asthma found that though ESS improved symptom scores, there was no observable improvement in pulmonary function [12].

In contrast, there is consistent evidence indicating that ESS can reduce dependency on asthma medications. Nishioka et al. in a 20-patient cohort found that patients reported reduced inhaler use and, among those using systemic medications for control of their asthma, 53.8% reported a reduction in systemic medication usage [130]. Dunlop and colleagues noted a 20% reduction in steroid inhaler usage and a significant reduction in oral steroid requirements in their study cohort of asthmatic CRS patients following ESS [135]. In a large cohort of 120 patients with CRS and concomitant asthma, ESS produced an approximate 50% reduction in inhaler usage and a nearly two-third decrease in oral steroid use over an average of 6.5 years [132]. Nishioka et al., in the same cohort reported above, found that 75% of patients noted a reduction in the number of ER and urgent care visits [130]. This was confirmed in two systematic reviews that demonstrated a trend toward fewer hospitalizations following ESS in patients with CRSwNP and concurrent asthma [136, 137].

Overall, ESS appears to be highly beneficial in patients with CRS who also have concurrent asthma, not only improving their sinus symptoms but also producing a generally reliable increase in asthma control, measured through QOL instruments and on pulmonary function testing, as well as reduced reliance on medications and fewer hospitalizations.

Aspirin Sensitivity

Both aspirin desensitization and ESS are critical components of AERD management and essential to long-term symptom control. Single-modality treatment can result in a failure rate as high as 90% [35, 138]. Current treatment recommendations suggest performing ESS followed by aspirin desensitization and therapy postoperatively [29]. It has been well established that aspirin desensitization improves overall symptoms and QOL [139–141]. McMains et al. found that there was a decreased likelihood of revision surgery in patients with AERD who underwent aspirin desensitization in addition to ESS [142]. However, some patients are intolerant to aspirin therapy, eliminating this as an option for treatment. Shah et al. found that ESS, in patients with AERD, enhances aspirin tolerance and that ESS can effectively convert patients who were aspirin intolerant prior to surgery to an aspirin-tolerant phenotype postoperatively, thereby allowing these patients to gain the advantages of long-term aspirin therapy [21].

The true impact of ESS on medical comorbidities in patients with AERD is best characterized when used in conjunction with aspirin therapy, as this is the optimal scenario based on the understanding of disease management. ESS has been found to enhance aspirin treatment response in patients with AERD when performed 3–6 weeks before initiation of aspirin desensitization and treatment [29]. Jerschow et al. found in 28 patients with AERD that ESS resulted in decreased aspirin sensitivity compared to baseline, with 12 of 28 patients having no reaction at all. Furthermore, there were lower urinary leukotriene E4 levels and a lower plasma prostaglandin D2-to-prostaglandin E2 ratio, indicating a mitigated reaction to aspirin [30]. Huang et al. noted similar results and noted that there was a statistically significant increase in aspirin-induced change in FEV_1 of almost 50% in patients who underwent ESS compared to those who did not. Moreover, they noted that there was a statistically significant decrease in both upper and lower airway reactions in patients who underwent ESS compared to those who did not [30, 143].

Patients with AERD have an overall improvement in their quality of life after ESS, which increases with a more complete approach to ESS versus a limited sinus-targeted approach and with the addition of aspirin treatment [99, 144]. In a retrospective review, Adappa et al. found a significant improvement in overall SNOT-22 scores in patients with AERD who underwent ESS followed by aspirin desensitization [29]. A systematic review of the role of surgical management of patients with AERD showed that most studies demonstrated improvement in sinus- and asthma-related symptoms as well as QOL measures after surgery [36].

Case Presentation

A 35-year-old male presented to the rhinology clinic with a history of AERD, diagnosed at an outside tertiary academic center through aspirin challenge, for which he had undergone 12 prior sinus surgeries. Each of these surgeries had produced only a transient symptom benefit. The patient had been intolerant of aspirin therapy due to gastrointestinal side effects and easy bruising on a maintenance dose of 650 mg twice daily.

At the time of presentation, the patient had bilateral nasal obstruction, chronic anterior and postnasal drainage, severe hyposmia, and bilateral cheek and forehead pressure. Nasal endoscopy indicated the presence of obstructive nasal polyps filling the middle meatus and extending into the sphenoethmoid recess bilaterally.

Initial medical management consisted of budesonide nasal rinses, a prednisone taper, and a 3-week course of clarithromycin followed by a CT sinus 1 month later (Fig. 6.1). The patient remained symptomatic and was deemed a candidate for a revision endoscopic sinus surgery including bilateral endoscopic maxillary mega-antrostomy, total ethmoidectomy, sphenoidotomy, and an EMLP (Fig. 6.2).

Three weeks postoperatively, the patient underwent single-day aspirin desensitization and was rapidly tapered to a 325 mg daily dose. He has tolerated this dose well without notable side effects. Furthermore, the patient was also started on dupilumab and maintained on 300 mg subcutaneous administration every 2 weeks.

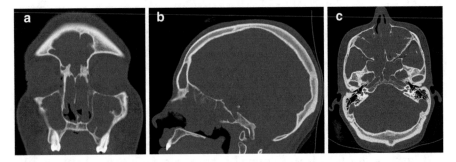

Fig. 6.1 High-resolution CT sinus without contrast in the (**a**) coronal, (**b**) sagittal, and (**c**) axial planes demonstrates total opacification of all right paranasal sinuses and evidence of prior endoscopic sinus surgery

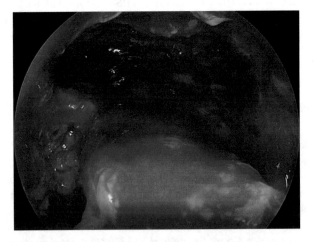

Fig. 6.2 Intraoperative 30° endoscopic view of the frontal ostium after EMLP following removal of the frontal sinus floor bilaterally, anterior to the middle turbinates, as well as superior and intersinus septectomy creating a large common drainage pathway for the paired frontal sinuses

Fig. 6.3 Postoperative 30° endoscopic view of the EMLP ostium at 6 months postoperatively. The patient is on aspirin maintenance therapy (325 mg daily) and regular dupilumab (300 mg every 2 weeks). There is wide patency of the contiguous bilateral frontal ostia and no evidence of nasal polyposis

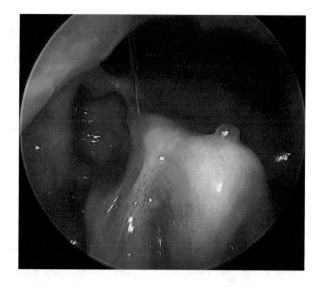

At 6 months postoperatively, the patient remained polyp-free and asymptomatic with no evidence of polyposis and a widely patent EMLP ostium (Fig. 6.3). At 24 months postoperatively, the patient remains polyp- and symptom-free.

Conclusion

When appropriate medical therapy fails, ESS and extended ESS are very effective for decreasing symptoms, improving quality-of-life scores, and managing patients with CRS with asthma or AERD. Postoperative maintenance therapies such as corticosteroid irrigation are critical for continued treatment of the underlying disease process and are synergistic with ESS. Additional benefits of ESS include improvement of cardinal symptoms, depression, and total economic burden. ESS also improves concomitant symptoms of asthma and enhances response to and facilitates aspirin desensitization in patients with AERD. ESS is essential for the treatment of CRS and asthma or AERD in patients who are recalcitrant to appropriate medical therapy.

References

1. Bresciani M, et al. Rhinosinusitis in severe asthma. J Allergy Clin Immunol. 2001;107(1):73–80.
2. Liou A, et al. Causative and contributive factors to asthma severity and patterns of medication use in patients seeking specialized asthma care. Chest. 2003;124(5):1781–8.

3. Palmer JN, et al. A cross-sectional, population-based survey of U.S. adults with symptoms of chronic rhinosinusitis. Allergy Asthma Proc. 2019;40(1):48–56.
4. Ek A, et al. Chronic rhinosinusitis in asthma is a negative predictor of quality of life: results from the Swedish GA(2)LEN survey. Allergy. 2013;68(10):1314–21.
5. Hamilos DL. Chronic rhinosinusitis: epidemiology and medical management. J Allergy Clin Immunol. 2011;128(4):693–707; quiz 708-9
6. Rajan JP, et al. Prevalence of aspirin-exacerbated respiratory disease among asthmatic patients: a meta-analysis of the literature. J Allergy Clin Immunol. 2015;135(3):676–81.. e1
7. Deal RT, Kountakis SE. Significance of nasal polyps in chronic rhinosinusitis: symptoms and surgical outcomes. Laryngoscope. 2004;114(11):1932–5.
8. Dufour X, et al. Diffuse nasal polyposis and endonasal endoscopic surgery: long-term results, a 65-case study. Laryngoscope. 2004;114(11):1982–7.
9. Rudmik L, et al. Defining appropriateness criteria for endoscopic sinus surgery during management of uncomplicated adult chronic rhinosinusitis: a RAND/UCLA appropriateness study. Rhinology. 2016;54(2):117–28.
10. Marambaia PP, et al. Use of the long-term quality of life assessment in the decision to indicate surgery in patients with chronic rhinosinusitis. Braz J Otorhinolaryngol. 2019;85(4):416–21.
11. Schlosser RJ, et al. Asthma quality of life and control after sinus surgery in patients with chronic rhinosinusitis. Allergy. 2017;72(3):483–91.
12. Chen FH, et al. Long-term results of endoscopic sinus surgery-oriented treatment for chronic rhinosinusitis with asthma. Laryngoscope. 2014;124(1):24–8.
13. Hopkins C, Andrews P, Holy CE. Does time to endoscopic sinus surgery impact outcomes in chronic rhinosinusitis? Retrospective analysis using the UK clinical practice research data. Rhinology. 2015;53(1):18–24.
14. Hopkins C, Rimmer J, Lund VJ. Does time to endoscopic sinus surgery impact outcomes in chronic rhinosinusitis? Prospective findings from the national comparative audit of surgery for nasal polyposis and chronic rhinosinusitis. Rhinology. 2015;53(1):10–7.
15. Soler ZM, et al. Cluster analysis and prediction of treatment outcomes for chronic rhinosinusitis. J Allergy Clin Immunol. 2016;137(4):1054–62.
16. Hopkins C, Rudmik L, Lund VJ. The predictive value of the preoperative sinonasal outcome test-22 score in patients undergoing endoscopic sinus surgery for chronic rhinosinusitis. Laryngoscope. 2015;125(8):1779–84.
17. Smith TL, et al. Medical therapy vs surgery for chronic rhinosinusitis: a prospective, multi-institutional study. Int Forum Allergy Rhinol. 2011;1(4):235–41.
18. Smith TL, et al. Medical therapy vs surgery for chronic rhinosinusitis: a prospective, multi-institutional study with 1-year follow-up. Int Forum Allergy Rhinol. 2013;3(1):4–9.
19. McFadden EA, et al. Surgery for sinusitis and aspirin triad. Laryngoscope. 1990;100(10 Pt 1):1043–6.
20. Batra PS, et al. Outcome analysis of endoscopic sinus surgery in patients with nasal polyps and asthma. Laryngoscope. 2003;113(10):1703–6.
21. Shah SJ, et al. Endoscopic sinus surgery improves aspirin treatment response in aspirin-exacerbated respiratory disease patients. Int Forum Allergy Rhinol. 2019;9(12):1401–8.
22. Wofford MR, et al. A computational study of functional endoscopic sinus surgery and maxillary sinus drug delivery. Rhinology. 2015;53(1):41–8.
23. Kumar H, Jain R. Review: the role of computational simulation in understanding the postoperative sinonasal environment. Clin Biomech (Bristol, Avon). 2019;66:2–10.
24. Grobler A, et al. Pre- and postoperative sinus penetration of nasal irrigation. Laryngoscope. 2008;118(11):2078–81.
25. Ragab SM, Lund VJ, Scadding G. Evaluation of the medical and surgical treatment of chronic rhinosinusitis: a prospective, randomised, controlled trial. Laryngoscope. 2004;114(5):923–30.
26. Orlandi RR, et al. International consensus statement on allergy and rhinology: rhinosinusitis. Int Forum Allergy Rhinol. 2016;6(Suppl 1):S22–209.

27. Kohanski MA, Toskala E, Kennedy DW. Evolution in the surgical management of chronic rhinosinusitis: current indications and pitfalls. J Allergy Clin Immunol. 2018;141(5):1561–9.
28. Awad OG, et al. Sinonasal outcomes after endoscopic sinus surgery in asthmatic patients with nasal polyps: a difference between aspirin-tolerant and aspirin-induced asthma? Laryngoscope. 2008;118(7):1282–6.
29. Adappa ND, et al. Outcomes after complete endoscopic sinus surgery and aspirin desensitization in aspirin-exacerbated respiratory disease. Int Forum Allergy Rhinol. 2018;8(1):49–53.
30. Jerschow E, et al. Sinus surgery is associated with a decrease in aspirin-induced reaction severity in patients with aspirin exacerbated respiratory disease. J Allergy Clin Immunol Pract. 2019;7(5):1580–8.
31. Philpott CM, et al. Endoscopic frontal sinusotomy-preventing recurrence or a route to revision? Laryngoscope. 2010;120(8):1682–6.
32. Kerrebijn JD, et al. If functional sinus surgery fails: a radical approach to sinus surgery. Otolaryngol Head Neck Surg. 1996;114(6):745–7.
33. Bassiouni A, Naidoo Y, Wormald PJ. When FESS fails: the inflammatory load hypothesis in refractory chronic rhinosinusitis. Laryngoscope. 2012;122(2):460–6.
34. Li KL, Lee AY, Abuzeid WM. Aspirin exacerbated respiratory disease: epidemiology, pathophysiology, and management. Med Sci (Basel). 2019;7(3):45.
35. Mendelsohn D, et al. Revision rates after endoscopic sinus surgery: a recurrence analysis. Ann Otol Rhinol Laryngol. 2011;120(3):162–6.
36. Adelman J, et al. The role of surgery in management of Samter's triad: a systematic review. Otolaryngol Head Neck Surg. 2016;155(2):220–37.
37. Szczeklik A, Nizankowska E. Clinical features and diagnosis of aspirin induced asthma. Thorax. 2000;55(Suppl 2):S42–4.
38. Young J, et al. Long-term outcome analysis of endoscopic sinus surgery for chronic sinusitis. Am J Rhinol. 2007;21(6):743–7.
39. Amar YG, Frenkiel S, Sobol SE. Outcome analysis of endoscopic sinus surgery for chronic sinusitis in patients having Samter's triad. J Otolaryngol. 2000;29(1):7–12.
40. Buras M, Simoncini A, Gungor A. Auto-obliteration of maxillary sinuses through osteoneogenesis in children with cystic fibrosis: a possible new way to reduce morbidity. Am J Otolaryngol. 2018;39(5):737–40.
41. Friedman WH, Katsantonis GP. Transantral revision of recurrent maxillary and ethmoidal disease following functional intranasal surgery. Otolaryngol Head Neck Surg. 1992;106(4):367–71.
42. Cho DY, Hwang PH. Results of endoscopic maxillary mega-antrostomy in recalcitrant maxillary sinusitis. Am J Rhinol. 2008;22(6):658–62.
43. Costa ML, et al. Long-term outcomes of endoscopic maxillary mega-antrostomy for refractory chronic maxillary sinusitis. Int Forum Allergy Rhinol. 2015;5(1):60–5.
44. Jankowski R, et al. Updating nasalisation: from concept to technique and results. Eur Ann Otorhinolaryngol Head Neck Dis. 2018;135(5):327–34.
45. Jankowski R, et al. Comparison of radical (nasalisation) and functional ethmoidectomy in patients with severe sinonasal polyposis. A retrospective study. Rev Laryngol Otol Rhinol (Bord). 2006;127(3):131–40.
46. Nguyen DT, Nguyen-Thi PL, Jankowski R. How does measured olfactory function correlate with self-ratings of the sense of smell in patients with nasal polyposis? Laryngoscope. 2012;122(5):947–52.
47. Leight WD, Leopold DA. Sphenoid "drill-out" for chronic sphenoid rhinosinusitis. Int Forum Allergy Rhinol. 2011;1(1):64–9.
48. Soler ZM, Sindwani R, Metson R. Endoscopic sphenoid nasalization for the treatment of advanced sphenoid disease. Otolaryngol Head Neck Surg. 2010;143(3):456–8.
49. Minni A, et al. Use of balloon catheter dilation and steroid-eluting stent in light and severe rhinosinusitis of frontal sinus: a multicenter retrospective randomized study. Eur Rev Med Pharmacol Sci. 2018;22(21):7482–91.

50. Naidoo Y, et al. Risk factors and outcomes for primary, revision, and modified Lothrop (Draf III) frontal sinus surgery. Int Forum Allergy Rhinol. 2013;3(5):412–7.
51. Chandra RK, et al. Factors associated with failure of frontal sinusotomy in the early follow-up period. Otolaryngol Head Neck Surg. 2004;131(4):514–8.
52. Abuzeid WM, et al. Endoscopic modified Lothrop procedure after failure of primary endoscopic sinus surgery: a meta-analysis. Int Forum Allergy Rhinol. 2018;8(5):605–13.
53. Patel VS, et al. Equivalence in outcomes between Draf 2B vs Draf 3 frontal sinusotomy for refractory chronic frontal rhinosinusitis. Int Forum Allergy Rhinol. 2018;8(1):25–31.
54. DeConde AS, et al. Prevalence of polyp recurrence after endoscopic sinus surgery for chronic rhinosinusitis with nasal polyposis. Laryngoscope. 2017;127(3):550–5.
55. Jang DW, et al. Aspirin sensitivity does not compromise quality-of-life outcomes in patients with Samter's triad. Laryngoscope. 2014;124(1):34–7.
56. Bassiouni A, Wormald PJ. Role of frontal sinus surgery in nasal polyp recurrence. Laryngoscope. 2013;123(1):36–41.
57. Morrissey DK, et al. Outcomes of modified endoscopic Lothrop in aspirin-exacerbated respiratory disease with nasal polyposis. Int Forum Allergy Rhinol. 2016;6(8):820–5.
58. Georgalas C, et al. Long terms results of Draf type III (modified endoscopic Lothrop) frontal sinus drainage procedure in 122 patients: a single centre experience. Rhinology. 2011;49(2):195–201.
59. Ye T, et al. Frontal ostium neo-osteogenesis and patency after Draf III procedure: a computer-assisted study. Int Forum Allergy Rhinol. 2014;4(9):739–44.
60. Schlosser RJ, et al. The endoscopic modified Lothrop: long-term follow-up on 44 patients. Am J Rhinol. 2002;16(2):103–8.
61. Conger BT Jr, Riley K, Woodworth BA. The Draf III mucosal grafting technique: a prospective study. Otolaryngol Head Neck Surg. 2012;146(4):664–8.
62. Rotenberg BW, et al. Postoperative care for Samter's triad patients undergoing endoscopic sinus surgery: a double-blinded, randomized controlled trial. Laryngoscope. 2011;121(12):2702–5.
63. Chen XZ, et al. The effects of nasal irrigation with various solutions after endoscopic sinus surgery: systematic review and meta-analysis. J Laryngol Otol. 2018;132(8):673–9.
64. Subramanian HN, Schechtman KB, Hamilos DL. A retrospective analysis of treatment outcomes and time to relapse after intensive medical treatment for chronic sinusitis. Am J Rhinol. 2002;16(6):303–12.
65. Farag AA, et al. Single-blind randomized controlled trial of surfactant vs hypertonic saline irrigation following endoscopic endonasal surgery. Int Forum Allergy Rhinol. 2013;3(4):276–80.
66. Achilles N, Mosges R. Nasal saline irrigations for the symptoms of acute and chronic rhinosinusitis. Curr Allergy Asthma Rep. 2013;13(2):229–35.
67. Liang KL, et al. Impact of pulsatile nasal irrigation on the prognosis of functional endoscopic sinus surgery. J Otolaryngol Head Neck Surg. 2008;37(2):148–53.
68. Talbot AR, Herr TM, Parsons DS. Mucociliary clearance and buffered hypertonic saline solution. Laryngoscope. 1997;107(4):500–3.
69. Principi N, Esposito S. Nasal irrigation: an imprecisely defined medical procedure. Int J Environ Res Public Health. 2017;14(5):516.
70. Naraghi M, et al. Improvement of sinonasal mucociliary function by endoscopic sinus surgery in patients with chronic rhinosinusitis. Am J Otolaryngol. 2018;39(6):707–10.
71. Harvey RJ, et al. Effects of endoscopic sinus surgery and delivery device on cadaver sinus irrigation. Otolaryngol Head Neck Surg. 2008;139(1):137–42.
72. Olson DE, Rasgon BM, Hilsinger RL Jr. Radiographic comparison of three methods for nasal saline irrigation. Laryngoscope. 2002;112(8 Pt 1):1394–8.
73. Pynnonen MA, et al. Nasal saline for chronic sinonasal symptoms: a randomized controlled trial. Arch Otolaryngol Head Neck Surg. 2007;133(11):1115–20.

74. Salib RJ, et al. A prospective randomised single-blinded clinical trial comparing the efficacy and tolerability of the nasal douching products Sterimar and Sinus Rinse following functional endoscopic sinus surgery. Clin Otolaryngol. 2013;38(4):297–305.
75. Gantz O, et al. Sinus irrigation penetration after balloon sinuplasty vs functional endoscopic sinus surgery in a cadaveric model. Int Forum Allergy Rhinol. 2019;9(9):953–7.
76. Craig JR, et al. Cadaveric validation study of computational fluid dynamics model of sinus irrigations before and after sinus surgery. Int Forum Allergy Rhinol. 2016;6(4):423–8.
77. Singhal D, et al. Effect of head position and surgical dissection on sinus irrigant penetration in cadavers. Laryngoscope. 2010;120(12):2528–31.
78. Zhao K, et al. Sinus irrigations before and after surgery-visualization through computational fluid dynamics simulations. Laryngoscope. 2016;126(3):E90–6.
79. Craig JR, Palmer JN, Zhao K. Computational fluid dynamic modeling of nose-to-ceiling head positioning for sphenoid sinus irrigation. Int Forum Allergy Rhinol. 2017;7(5):474–9.
80. Inthavong K, et al. Characterization of nasal irrigation flow from a squeeze bottle using computational fluid dynamics. Int Forum Allergy Rhinol. 2020;10(1):29–40.
81. Govindaraju R, et al. Extent of maxillary sinus surgery and its effect on instrument access, irrigation penetration, and disease clearance. Int Forum Allergy Rhinol. 2019;9(10):1097–104.
82. Snidvongs K, et al. Sinus surgery and delivery method influence the effectiveness of topical corticosteroids for chronic rhinosinusitis: systematic review and meta-analysis. Am J Rhinol Allergy. 2013;27(3):221–33.
83. Lildholdt T, Rundcrantz H, Lindqvist N. Efficacy of topical corticosteroid powder for nasal polyps: a double-blind, placebo-controlled study of budesonide. Clin Otolaryngol Allied Sci. 1995;20(1):26–30.
84. Snidvongs K, et al. Topical steroid for chronic rhinosinusitis without polyps. Cochrane Database Syst Rev. 2011;8:CD009274.
85. Snidvongs K, et al. Corticosteroid nasal irrigations after endoscopic sinus surgery in the management of chronic rhinosinusitis. Int Forum Allergy Rhinol. 2012;2(5):415–21.
86. Huang ZZ, et al. Budesonide nasal irrigation improved Lund-Kennedy endoscopic score of chronic rhinosinusitis patients after endoscopic sinus surgery. Eur Arch Otorhinolaryngol. 2019;276(5):1397–403.
87. Joe SA, Thambi R, Huang J. A systematic review of the use of intranasal steroids in the treatment of chronic rhinosinusitis. Otolaryngol Head Neck Surg. 2008;139(3):340–7.
88. Harvey RJ, et al. Corticosteroid nasal irrigations are more effective than simple sprays in a randomized double-blinded placebo-controlled trial for chronic rhinosinusitis after sinus surgery. Int Forum Allergy Rhinol. 2018;8(4):461–70.
89. Harvey RJ, et al. Fluid residuals and drug exposure in nasal irrigation. Otolaryngol Head Neck Surg. 2009;141(6):757–61.
90. Neubauer PD, Schwam ZG, Manes RP. Comparison of intranasal fluticasone spray, budesonide atomizer, and budesonide respules in patients with chronic rhinosinusitis with polyposis after endoscopic sinus surgery. Int Forum Allergy Rhinol. 2016;6(3):233–7.
91. Lindqvist N, et al. Long-term safety and efficacy of budesonide nasal aerosol in perennial rhinitis. A 12-month multicentre study. Allergy. 1986;41(3):179–86.
92. Pipkorn U, et al. Long-term safety of budesonide nasal aerosol: a 5.5-year follow-up study. Clin Allergy. 1988;18(3):253–9.
93. Soudry E, et al. Safety analysis of long-term budesonide nasal irrigations in patients with chronic rhinosinusitis post endoscopic sinus surgery. Int Forum Allergy Rhinol. 2016;6(6):568–72.
94. Yoon HY, et al. Post-operative corticosteroid irrigation for chronic rhinosinusitis after endoscopic sinus surgery: a meta-analysis. Clin Otolaryngol. 2018;43(2):525–32.
95. Patel ZM, et al. Surgical therapy vs continued medical therapy for medically refractory chronic rhinosinusitis: a systematic review and meta-analysis. Int Forum Allergy Rhinol. 2017;7(2):119–27.

96. Smith KA, et al. Endoscopic sinus surgery compared to continued medical therapy for patients with refractory chronic rhinosinusitis. Int Forum Allergy Rhinol. 2014;4(10):823–7.
97. Smith TL, et al. Determinants of outcomes of sinus surgery: a multi-institutional prospective cohort study. Otolaryngol Head Neck Surg. 2010;142(1):55–63.
98. Smith TL, et al. Long-term outcomes of endoscopic sinus surgery in the management of adult chronic rhinosinusitis. Int Forum Allergy Rhinol. 2019;9(8):831–41.
99. DeConde AS, et al. Outcomes of complete vs targeted approaches to endoscopic sinus surgery. Int Forum Allergy Rhinol. 2015;5(8):691–700.
100. Abuzeid WM, et al. Outcomes of chronic frontal sinusitis treated with ethmoidectomy: a prospective study. Int Forum Allergy Rhinol. 2016;6(6):597–604.
101. Chester AC, Antisdel JL, Sindwani R. Symptom-specific outcomes of endoscopic sinus surgery: a systematic review. Otolaryngol Head Neck Surg. 2009;140(5):633–9.
102. DeConde AS, et al. Investigation of change in cardinal symptoms of chronic rhinosinusitis after surgical or ongoing medical management. Int Forum Allergy Rhinol. 2015;5(1):36–45.
103. Van Gerven L, et al. Lack of long-term add-on effect by montelukast in postoperative chronic rhinosinusitis patients with nasal polyps. Laryngoscope. 2018;128(8):1743–51.
104. Briner HR, Jones N, Simmen D. Olfaction after endoscopic sinus surgery: long-term results. Rhinology. 2012;50(2):178–84.
105. Oka H, et al. Olfactory changes after endoscopic sinus surgery in patients with chronic rhinosinusitis. Auris Nasus Larynx. 2013;40(5):452–7.
106. Gupta D, et al. Impact of endoscopic sinus surgery on olfaction and use of alternative components in odor threshold measurement. Am J Rhinol Allergy. 2015;29(4):e117–20.
107. Gudziol V, et al. Olfaction and sinonasal symptoms in patients with CRSwNP and AERD and without AERD: a cross-sectional and longitudinal study. Eur Arch Otorhinolaryngol. 2017;274(3):1487–93.
108. Soler ZM, et al. Olfactory-specific quality of life outcomes after endoscopic sinus surgery. Int Forum Allergy Rhinol. 2016;6(4):407–13.
109. Zi XX, et al. Olfactory change pattern after endoscopic sinus surgery in chronic rhinosinusitis with olfactory dysfunction. J Coll Physicians Surg Pak. 2018;28(8):612–7.
110. Wong EH, et al. Patient-reported olfaction improves following outside-in Draf III frontal sinus surgery for chronic rhinosinusitis. Laryngoscope. 2019;129(1):25–30.
111. Katotomichelakis M, et al. Olfactory dysfunction and asthma as risk factors for poor quality of life in upper airway diseases. Am J Rhinol Allergy. 2013;27(4):293–8.
112. Kohli P, et al. Olfactory outcomes after endoscopic sinus surgery for chronic rhinosinusitis: a meta-analysis. Otolaryngol Head Neck Surg. 2016;155(6):936–48.
113. Kern RC. Chronic sinusitis and anosmia: pathologic changes in the olfactory mucosa. Laryngoscope. 2000;110(7):1071–7.
114. Schlosser RJ, et al. Burden of illness: a systematic review of depression in chronic rhinosinusitis. Am J Rhinol Allergy. 2016;30(4):250–6.
115. Katotomichelakis M, et al. Demographic correlates of anxiety and depression symptoms in chronic sinonasal diseases. Int J Psychiatry Med. 2014;48(2):83–94.
116. Litvack JR, Mace J, Smith TL. Role of depression in outcomes of endoscopic sinus surgery. Otolaryngol Head Neck Surg. 2011;144(3):446–51.
117. Schlosser RJ, et al. Depression-specific outcomes after treatment of chronic rhinosinusitis. JAMA Otolaryngol Head Neck Surg. 2016;142(4):370–6.
118. Alt JA, et al. Sleep quality outcomes after medical and surgical management of chronic rhinosinusitis. Int Forum Allergy Rhinol. 2017;7(2):113–8.
119. Adams KN, et al. Self-reported anxiety and depression unchanged after endoscopic sinus surgery for chronic rhinosinusitis. Rhinology. 2018;56(3):234–40.
120. Ospina J, et al. The impact of comorbid depression in chronic rhinosinusitis on post-operative sino-nasal quality of life and pain following endoscopic sinus surgery. J Otolaryngol Head Neck Surg. 2019;48(1):18.

121. Caulley L, et al. Direct costs of adult chronic rhinosinusitis by using 4 methods of estimation: results of the US medical expenditure panel survey. J Allergy Clin Immunol. 2015;136(6):1517–22.
122. Smith KA, Orlandi RR, Rudmik L. Cost of adult chronic rhinosinusitis: a systematic review. Laryngoscope. 2015;125(7):1547–56.
123. Scangas GA, et al. Cost utility analysis of endoscopic sinus surgery for chronic rhinosinusitis. Int Forum Allergy Rhinol. 2016;6(6):582–9.
124. Scangas GA, et al. The impact of asthma on the cost effectiveness of surgery for chronic rhinosinusitis with nasal polyps. Int Forum Allergy Rhinol. 2017;7(11):1035–44.
125. Rudmik L, et al. Productivity costs decrease after endoscopic sinus surgery for refractory chronic rhinosinusitis. Laryngoscope. 2016;126(3):570–4.
126. Rudmik L, et al. Economic evaluation of endoscopic sinus surgery versus continued medical therapy for refractory chronic rhinosinusitis. Laryngoscope. 2015;125(1):25–32.
127. Ehnhage A, et al. Functional endoscopic sinus surgery improved asthma symptoms as well as PEFR and olfaction in patients with nasal polyposis. Allergy. 2009;64(5):762–9.
128. Ehnhage A, et al. One year after endoscopic sinus surgery in polyposis: asthma, olfaction, and quality-of-life outcomes. Otolaryngol Head Neck Surg. 2012;146(5):834–41.
129. Olsson P, et al. Quality of life is improved by endoscopic surgery and fluticasone in nasal polyposis with asthma. Rhinology. 2010;48(3):325–30.
130. Nishioka GJ, et al. Functional endoscopic sinus surgery in patients with chronic sinusitis and asthma. Otolaryngol Head Neck Surg. 1994;110(6):494–500.
131. Dunlop G, Scadding GK, Lund VJ. The effect of endoscopic sinus surgery on asthma: management of patients with chronic rhinosinusitis, nasal polyposis, and asthma. Am J Rhinol. 1999;13(4):261–5.
132. Senior BA, et al. Long-term impact of functional endoscopic sinus surgery on asthma. Otolaryngol Head Neck Surg. 1999;121(1):66–8.
133. Dejima K, et al. A clinical study of endoscopic sinus surgery for sinusitis in patients with bronchial asthma. Int Arch Allergy Immunol. 2005;138(2):97–104.
134. Ikeda K, et al. Endoscopic sinus surgery improves pulmonary function in patients with asthma associated with chronic sinusitis. Ann Otol Rhinol Laryngol. 1999;108(4):355–9.
135. Dunlop W, Heron L, Fox G, Greaney M. Budget impact analysis of a fixed-dose combination of fluticasone propionate and formoterol fumarate (FP/FORM) in a pressurized metered-dose inhaler (pMDI) for asthma. Adv Ther. 2013;30(10):933–44.
136. Vashishta R, et al. A systematic review and meta-analysis of asthma outcomes following endoscopic sinus surgery for chronic rhinosinusitis. Int Forum Allergy Rhinol. 2013;3(10):788–94.
137. Rix I, et al. Management of chronic rhinosinusitis with nasal polyps and coexisting asthma: a systematic review. Am J Rhinol Allergy. 2015;29(3):193–201.
138. Sakalar EG, et al. Aspirin-exacerbated respiratory disease and current treatment modalities. Eur Arch Otorhinolaryngol. 2017;274(3):1291–300.
139. Berges-Gimeno MP, Simon RA, Stevenson DD. Long-term treatment with aspirin desensitization in asthmatic patients with aspirin-exacerbated respiratory disease. J Allergy Clin Immunol. 2003;111(1):180–6.
140. Klimek L, Pfaar O. Aspirin intolerance: does desensitization alter the course of the disease? Immunol Allergy Clin N Am. 2009;29(4):669–75.
141. Lee RU, Stevenson DD. Aspirin-exacerbated respiratory disease: evaluation and management. Allergy Asthma Immunol Res. 2011;3(1):3–10.
142. McMains KC, Kountakis SE. Medical and surgical considerations in patients with Samter's triad. Am J Rhinol. 2006;20(6):573–6.
143. Huang GX, et al. Sinus surgery improves lower respiratory tract reactivity during aspirin desensitization for AERD. J Allergy Clin Immunol Pract. 2019;7(5):1647–9.
144. Cho KS, et al. Long-term sinonasal outcomes of aspirin desensitization in aspirin exacerbated respiratory disease. Otolaryngol Head Neck Surg. 2014;151(4):575–81.

Chapter 7
Aspirin-Exacerbated Respiratory Disease

Auddie M. Sweis and John V. Bosso

> **Key Concepts**
> - Aspirin-exacerbated respiratory disease (AERD) consists of asthma, eosinophilic CRS with nasal polyposis, and the development of respiratory reactions to COX-1 inhibitors.
> - Endoscopic sinus surgery, often including extended approaches, is central to treating AERD.
> - Aspirin desensitization, combined with surgical therapy, provides the optimal outcomes for controlling inflammatory symptoms in AERD patients.

Definition of Disorder

Aspirin-exacerbated respiratory disease (AERD), also referred to as Samter's triad or in Europe and the Middle East as NSAID-exacerbated respiratory disease (NERD), is a progressive, acquired syndrome that is non-IgE mediated. AERD consists of asthma, eosinophilic chronic rhinosinusitis with nasal polyposis, and the development of respiratory reactions to COX-1 inhibitors. Respiratory reactions involve the upper airways (i.e., nasal congestion, rhinorrhea, sneezing) and/or the lower airways (i.e., wheeze, shortness of breath, cough, chest tightness). Patients may also experience gastrointestinal symptoms (i.e., abdominal pain, nausea,

A. M. Sweis · J. V. Bosso (✉)
Division of Rhinology, Department of Otorhinolaryngology, Head and Neck Surgery,
Perelman School of Medicine, University of Pennsylvania, Philadelphia, PA, USA
e-mail: John.Bosso@pennmedicine.upenn.edu

© Springer Nature Switzerland AG 2020
D. A. Gudis, R. J. Schlosser (eds.), *The Unified Airway*,
https://doi.org/10.1007/978-3-030-50330-7_7

vomiting) and cutaneous symptoms (i.e., urticaria, rash, or angioedema). The consumption of alcoholic beverages also triggers upper and/or lower respiratory tract symptoms in 83% of AERD patients [1]. The peak onset of AERD occurs in the third and fourth decades of life and very rarely occurs before puberty [2, 3]. The condition is an aggressive inflammatory disorder of the sinuses and lower airways that progresses despite the avoidance of aspirin/NSAIDs [4].

Epidemiology

Stevenson et al. performed a meta-analysis which demonstrated that the prevalence of AERD was 7.2% in the general population of patients with asthma. The prevalence of asthma in the United States is 19 million. Coupling these two data points, the estimated prevalence of AERD in the United States is 1,368,000. Further analysis demonstrated that the prevalence of AERD was 14.9% in patients with severe asthma, 9.7% in patients with nasal polyps, and 8.7% in patients with chronic rhinosinusitis [5, 6]. In a retrospective analysis, Cahill et al. demonstrated that 12.4% of patients who met the criteria for an AERD diagnosis did not have a diagnosis of AERD in the medical record and were never referred for oral aspirin challenge or aspirin desensitization [7]. In essence, Cahill et al. demonstrate that the diagnosis of AERD can oftentimes be overlooked. Laidlaw et al. also emphasize the importance of early and proper diagnosis for three key reasons: (1) to educate patients on avoidance of medications that fall within the umbrella of COX-1 inhibitors so as to optimize patient safety, (2) to provide disease-tailored therapies, and (3) to educate AERD patients on alternative non-COX-1 pain relief medications to potentially decrease future overuse of opioids [8].

Etiology and Pathogenesis

In AERD, there is a constant inflammatory response within the respiratory mucosa characterized by mast cell activation, eosinophilic inflammation, and elevated leukotriene levels as well as receptors [9]. AERD possesses a unique inflammatory pathway, the hallmark being dysregulation of the 5-lipoxygenase-leukotriene C4 (LTC4) synthase pathway. Group 2 innate lymphoid cells (ILC2) reside at the mucosal surface and augment immune activation through the production of interleukin (IL) 4, IL-5, and IL-13 after stimulation by cytokines IL-25, IL-33, thymic stromal lymphopoietin (TSLP), prostaglandin D2 (PGD2), and cysteinyl leukotrienes (Fig. 7.1). This LTC4 synthase pathway converts arachidonic acid to the cysteinyl leukotrienes (LTC4/LTD4/LTE4). Leukotriene E4 (LTE4) is the stable end metabolite of the cysteinyl leukotrienes. It is cysteinyl leukotrienes that potently induce bronchoconstriction, vascular permeability, increased mucous secretion, and eosinophilic inflammation. Christie et al. demonstrated that the urinary levels of LTE4 in patients with AERD are higher than control patients, and these levels notably increase during NSAID-induced reactions [10]. Bosso et al. identified elevations in

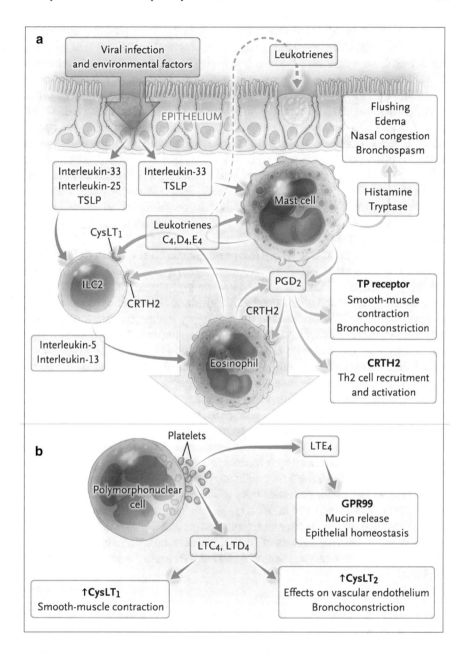

Fig. 7.1 Inflammatory pathways in AERD. (**a**) Type 2 inflammatory pathway seen in AERD patients. (**b**) Increased leukotriene levels in AERD patients secondary to platelet-adherent neutrophils

serum tryptase and plasma histamine levels during NSAID-induced reactions, further supporting the presence of mast cell activation in the inflammatory process of patients with AERD [11]. Wells et al. showed that mast cell-stabilizing drugs can block the increase in products of activated mast cells (e.g., histamine, PGD2, and

LTC4) that parallel NSAID-induced elevations in LTE4 in patients with AERD [12]. And so, mast cell activation is a key contributor to cysteinyl leukotriene formation during COX-1 inhibition in patients with AERD. Elevated cysteinyl leukotriene levels also occur because of a strong eosinophil overexpression of LTC4 synthase in bronchial biopsies of patients with AERD as compared to aspirin-tolerant patient controls. Additionally, the blood and sinonasal tissues of patients with AERD have an abnormally large number of platelet-adherent neutrophils, monocytes, and eosinophils. Platelets express LTC4 synthase and were noted to contribute to approximately 70% of cysteinyl leukotriene formation by adhering to 5-lipoxygenase-expressing granulocytes and promoting LTC4 synthesis via transmembrane transfer of metabolic intermediates. Serum levels of platelet-adherent granulocytes correlated strongly with basal levels of LTE4 in urine [13–16]. Together, these findings support the concept of dysregulation of the 5-lipoxygenase-LTC4 synthase pathway.

The literature supports the theory that prostaglandin E2 (PGE2), a COX pathway product, maintains homeostasis with regard to 5-lipoxygenase activity and mast cell activation. Normally, PGE2 is upregulated during periods of inflammation via expression of COX-2 and microsomal PGE2 synthase [17]. Studies suggest that the upregulation of PGE2 is impaired in the respiratory tissues in patients with AERD [18]. That is, in patients with AERD, the production of PGE2 may depend disproportionately on COX-1 and be especially susceptible to low levels when patients with AERD ingest COX-1 inhibitors. Predominantly, PGE2 signaling occurs through E prostanoid-2 receptors and ultimately prevents mast cell activation and inhibits 5-lipoxygenase function and platelet activation [19–22]. E prostanoid-2 receptor expression by mast cells, eosinophils, neutrophils, and T cells within the respiratory mucosa has been shown to be diminished in patients with AERD [23]. This decreased receptor expression has been demonstrated to be under epigenetic control, potentially influenced by infections or exposure to environmental allergens [24]. Stevenson et al. showed that childhood exposure to environmental tobacco smoke is associated with increased odds of developing AERD, further promoting the involvement of epigenetics in AERD [25]. Van Sambeek et al. conducted molecular biological assays in an attempt to correlate promoter gene alleles for leukotriene C4 synthase with a diagnosis of AERD; however, no correlation was identified [26]. Overall, the current literature on AERD argues against a strong genetic basis for AERD.

Clinical Presentation

Patient Demographic and Medical Context

The peak onset of AERD is in the third to fourth decade of life with a slight predilection toward females [3]. Rarely, AERD occurs in younger patients. Black and Latino patients with AERD have been reported to have more severe respiratory reactions to COX-1 inhibitors than white patients [27]. AERD is prevalent throughout the world; however, the prevalence in China is reported at only 0.57% [28]. No familial patterns exist. It has been demonstrated that a history of atopy, described as positive IgE skin or in vitro testing to common aeroallergens, coexists in approximately 66% of patients with AERD [2, 29].

Signs and Symptoms

Patients with AERD have chronic symptoms of asthma and rhinosinusitis. These symptoms may include persistent coughing, wheezing, chest tightness, shortness of breath, anosmia, postnasal drip, anterior rhinorrhea, and facial pressure and pain. Patients typically then develop acute exacerbations of upper and lower airway symptoms after the ingestion of NSAIDs. Classical acute reactions include increased watery rhinorrhea, nasal congestion, and nasal obstruction; periorbital edema; conjunctival injection; and/or worsening dyspnea, chest tightness, and wheezing. A drop in the forced expiratory volume in 1 second (FEV1) typically occurs in conjunction with the lower airway symptoms. This bronchoconstriction is often reversible with an inhaled beta-agonist. The onset of symptoms on average occurs 30 minutes to 3 hours after the ingestion of NSAIDs [30]. The severity of symptoms has been shown to increase as the dose of NSAID ingestion increases [29]. Ta et al. demonstrate that the majority of patients with AERD reported a diminished quality of life mainly because of chronic nasal symptoms and hyposmia. Most patients with AERD also describe an exacerbation of upper and lower airway reactions after the ingestion of alcohol [1, 31].

The average time frame for the development of AERD is over the course of several years. Most patients, often in their third to fourth decade of life, develop persistent rhinitis despite appropriate medical therapy. Subsequently, patients begin to experience nasal congestion and anosmia and develop nasal polyps all secondary to eosinophilic rhinosinusitis [3]. Usually, patients report a history of multiple sinus surgeries and/or polypectomies. Lower airway symptoms almost always develop as chronic rhinosinusitis worsens. Sometimes, the onset of asthma will antedate the upper respiratory complaints. Typically, patients develop a sensitivity to aspirin/NSAIDs later during this progression of symptoms. Symptoms of asthma and chronic rhinosinusitis continue to worsen despite the avoidance of aspirin/NSAID products [2, 32, 33]. Upper airway symptoms, such as diminished sense of smell, have been shown to disrupt the quality of life of patients more so than lower airway symptoms [29].

In patients with AERD who have severe respiratory reactions to ingested NSAIDs, additional symptoms can occur and may include laryngospasm, abdominal pain, facial flushing, and hypotension. Moreover, 15% of AERD patients can have urticaria and/or angioedema during an acute respiratory reaction. This can at times be confused with isolated NSAID-induced urticaria or angioedema. The latter is NSAID sensitivity without respiratory reactions [34].

AERD patients may rarely report angina-like chest pain associated with marked peripheral blood eosinophilia. The pain is described as retrosternal and squeezing in quality, and it may radiate to the jaw, neck, or upper extremities. In this group of patients, other causes of chest pain have been ruled out, and the pain typically improves with systemic corticosteroids while not responding to nitrates [35].

Diagnostics

Typical Physical Exam/Nasal Endoscopy Findings with Figures

The diagnosis of AERD can be made clinically when the following three conditions are present: a history of asthma, the presence of chronic rhinosinusitis with nasal polyposis (Fig. 7.2), and a history of upper and/or lower respiratory reactions to NSAID ingestion. Rarely, clinical asthma or bronchial hyperreactivity is absent and the patient is identified as an upper airway variant of AERD. As many as 15% of patients with AERD are unable to identify whether or not they have respiratory reactions to COX-1 inhibitors. The majority of these patients report that they in fact have no adverse reactions to COX-1 inhibitors. It is in this subgroup of AERD patients that an aspirin challenge is required in order to make the proper diagnosis of AERD [32]. Another subgroup of AERD patients may not report any reactions to COX-1 inhibitors because they take a cardiovascular prophylactic aspirin 81 mg daily, essentially resulting in low-dose aspirin desensitization without necessarily being aware of it. If such desensitization is suspected, holding the aspirin for 10 days should be a sufficient window of time, after which exposure to aspirin will result in upper and lower

Fig. 7.2 Endoscopic view of nasal polyp

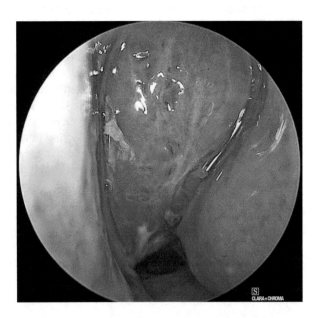

airway reactions [36]. Other patients who should undergo an aspirin challenge to aid in the diagnosis of AERD are patients who have not used NSAIDs recently, patients on leukotriene-modifying agents, and patients with severe asthma and nasal polyposis who may be less aware of respiratory reactions to NSAIDs [37, 38].

Patients with AERD will have reactions to all COX-1 inhibitors, not just one specific COX-1 inhibitor. In patients with a history of chronic rhinosinusitis with nasal polyps, asthma, and a history of a single NSAID reaction, there is an 80% likelihood of having a positive oral aspirin challenge. In patients with two or more reactions, the likelihood increases to 89% [39]. LTE4 is a stable end product of the cysteinyl leukotriene pathway. Measurement of its concentration in the urine as a marker of this pathway has been validated [40]. With regard to predicting a history of aspirin sensitivity prior to an aspirin challenge, the 24-hour urinary LTE4 level of 166 pg/mg Cr was noted to have a sensitivity of 76%, a specificity of 89%, and a negative predictive value of 97%; however, the positive predictive value is only 40% [41]. Furthermore, the test is not widely available. Therefore, even with this diagnostic test available, oral aspirin challenge still remains the gold standard for a definitive diagnosis of AERD.

Typical CT Radiographic Features with Figures

On computed tomography (CT), patients with AERD trend toward complete bilateral paranasal pan-sinus opacification (Fig. 7.3). Stevenson et al. showed 99% of patients with AERD have abnormal sinus opacification on CT [2]. Mascia et al. showed that AERD patients have worse Lund-Mackay scores compared to those without AERD, with a statistical significance of $p < 0.001$. A normal CT sinus essentially rules out AERD [42].

Medical Management and Outcomes

The concept of a unified airway guides the treatment options for patients with AERD. It is well known that patients with chronic rhinosinusitis (CRS) have better lower airway outcomes with improved management of their upper airway [43].

Systemic Medical Therapy

Systemic medical therapies include corticosteroids, leukotriene-modifying agents (LTMAs), aspirin therapy after desensitization (ATAD), and T2 biologics that target type 2 inflammatory cytokines.

A course of oral corticosteroids transiently reduces the upper and lower airway symptom scores and polyp size in patients with AERD. Therefore, oral corticosteroids may be used judiciously to help control exacerbations of upper and lower

Fig. 7.3 Computed
tomography demonstrating
complete opacification of
the sinuses bilaterally

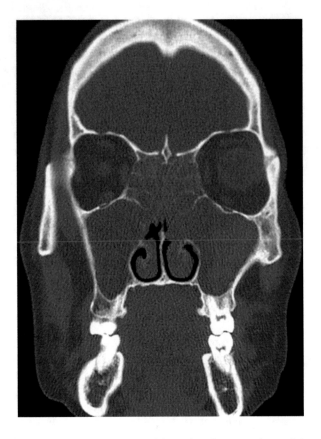

airway symptoms [44]. Oral antibiotics are an acceptable option for acute bacterial sinopulmonary infections. Though it has been demonstrated that patients with AERD-related CRSwNP have higher levels of staphylococcal enterotoxins when compared to patients with non-AERD CRSwNP, a clinical benefit from treating the former group with oral antistaphylococcal antibiotics has not been demonstrated [45]. Oral antihistamines may be beneficial to AERD patients with comorbid allergic rhinitis, particularly those with symptoms of sneezing and rhinorrhea [46]. Long-term oral alpha-adrenergic decongestants are not recommended due to the increased risk of hypertension. LTMAs currently include 5-lipoxygenase inhibitors (i.e., zileuton) and cysteinyl leukotriene-1 receptor blockers (i.e., montelukast or zafirlukast). Studies demonstrate that the addition of an LTMA to preexisting therapy for AERD helps improve upper and lower respiratory symptoms [47, 48]. For example, the addition of montelukast resulted in a 10% increase in forced expiratory volume in 1 second (FEV1), higher morning peak flow rates, decreased use of rescue medication, decreased number of asthma exacerbations, and a significant improvement in asthma quality-of-life scores. The addition of zileuton resulted in an improvement of pulmonary function tests and sinonasal quality-of-life scores and a decrease in the use of short-acting beta-agonists for symptom relief. As AERD patients may ultimately undergo oral aspirin challenge (OAC) and subsequent aspirin desensitization, LTMAs have the added benefit of reducing the severity of bronchospastic reactions during aspirin desensitization or during accidental exposure to aspirin or NSAIDs [49]. While LTMAs have been shown to control lower airway symptoms in AERD patients, Dahlin et al. demonstrated that zileuton also improved loss of sense of smell, nasal congestion, and rhinorrhea [47, 48]. In another study, Laidlaw et al. demonstrated that a subset of AERD patients receiving zileuton therapy had the greatest improvement in FEV1 [31, 50].

Avoidance of specific medications is central to preventing acute respiratory reactions. AERD patients who have not undergone aspirin desensitization should avoid all NSAIDs that inhibit COX-1. Highly selective COX-2 inhibitors have been shown to be safe for use in AERD patients [51]. While most AERD patients tolerate acetaminophen, approximately one-third of patients with AERD will have mild respiratory reactions when they ingest 1000 mg or greater of this analgesic likely due to its weak inhibition of COX-1 [52].

Beyond the above therapies described, at least 16 studies (four double-blind placebo-controlled) over the past three decades have supported aspirin desensitization as central to the management of AERD. Desensitization is indicated in patients with (1) persistent upper and lower airway symptoms despite appropriate medical therapy for asthma and appropriate medical and surgical therapy for CRSwNP, (2) AERD patients with comorbidities that would benefit from the use of aspirin and other NSAIDs (i.e., arthritis, coronary artery disease requiring antiplatelet therapy, etc.), (3) patients who require frequent bursts of systemic corticosteroids, and (4) patients with rapidly growing nasal polyps following ESS. Aspirin desensitization targets and suppresses the abnormal leukotriene metabolism that occurs in AERD patients, resulting in tolerance to aspirin and other NSAIDs. Walters et al. demonstrated that 85% of AERD patients who underwent desensitization 10 years prior and were compliant with ATAD reported persistent improvement in symptoms. Moreover, at 10 years out from desensitization, 62% of patients continued on with daily aspirin therapy due to the clinical benefit they reported, and 38% discontinued daily aspirin for a variety of reasons (i.e., lack of noticeable benefit, preparation for an upcoming surgery, or an adverse reaction to daily aspirin) [53]. Such findings have been corroborated by Berges-Gimeno et al. [2]. ATAD has been shown to slow the rate of nasal polyposis recurrence and reduce the need for repeat sinus surgery [54].

Prior to beginning aspirin desensitization, LTMAs can be started at least 3 days prior to and throughout the procedure. LTMAs have been shown to decrease lower airway symptoms while preserving upper airway symptoms during desensitization [37, 55, 47, 48]. If a patient is taking inhaled corticosteroids (ICS) and long-acting beta 2 agonists (LABA) prior to starting desensitization, these medications should be continued during desensitization. Like LTMA, ICSs and LABAs shift reactions to aspirin desensitization from the lower airway to the upper airway [56]. If patients have poorly controlled asthma prior to starting desensitization, it is imperative to improve control prior to the beginning. In such scenarios, patients may benefit from a course of oral corticosteroids. The role of oral antihistamines prior to aspirin desensitization remains unclear, as some believe it may blunt upper airway reactions to aspirin, while others have conducted aspirin desensitization without issue in patients on oral antihistamines [57, 58].

Aspirin desensitization can be completed in an outpatient setting (properly equipped for allergic emergencies) for most patients with AERD. Such patients should not be on beta-blockers, have well-controlled asthma, and lack any other notable comorbidities. Patients with poorly controlled asthma (FEV1 <70%) should undergo aspirin desensitization in an inpatient setting [59]. The standard US protocols for aspirin desensitization include the following: (1) a 2-day oral aspirin desensitization protocol, (2) a 2-day intranasal ketorolac plus oral aspirin desensitization protocol, and (3) a 1-day aspirin desensitization protocol (Table 7.1). Lee et al. demonstrated that the intranasal ketorolac protocol offers the benefit of an excellent safety profile, with an increased percentage of naso-ocular reactions during desensitization. The disadvantage is that intranasal ketorolac is not as readily available as oral aspirin [60].

Regardless of the protocol utilized, the standard maximum dose of aspirin during desensitization is 325 mg. Hope et al. demonstrated that if patients do not experience respiratory symptoms at 325 mg, they do not exhibit additional symptoms at higher doses [30]. The gold standard for diagnosis of AERD is the development of symptoms during an oral aspirin challenge. Patients typically have a decrease in their FEV1 by at least 15% or a reduction in peak nasal inspiratory flow (PNIF) by at least 20% [61]. Symptoms include upper and lower airway reactions, cutaneous symptoms, or gastrointestinal symptoms as previously reviewed. These symptoms usually self-resolve within 3–4 hours of onset. Typically, the dose around which symptoms are first noted is 60–80 mg of aspirin. All symptoms range from mild and transient to severe and persistent. If the latter, aspirin desensitization may need to be discontinued. Depending on the symptoms that arise, various treatment options exist. For nasal congestion, intranasal antihistamines, intranasal corticosteroids, intranasal decongestants, or oral antihistamines can be administered. Lower airway reactions can be managed with short-acting beta-agonists. Laryngeal reactions may be managed with inhaled racemic epinephrine. Gastrointestinal symptoms can be treated with H-2 blockers and/or antiemetics. Cutaneous symptoms can be treated with antihistamines. Multisystem or severe single system reactions should be treated with intramuscular epinephrine.

It is difficult to predict the severity of a patient's reaction to an oral aspirin challenge and/or aspirin desensitization. However, urine levels of LTE4 and PGD2, as previously discussed, correlate with the severity of respiratory reactions. Additionally, the following have been shown to impact the severity of symptoms during aspirin desensitization: (1) duration of the challenge; (2) the desensitization protocol utilized; (3) whether or not the patient has had sinus surgery (i.e., the current state of polyp burden); and (4) whether or not the patient is on LTMAs, antihistamines, or mast cell stabilizers [34, 37, 56]. Risk factors that are associated with a positive oral aspirin challenge include FEV1 <80% predicted, the lack of LTMA use during the time of challenge, and a history of asthma exacerbations requiring emergency room visits [39]. Risk factors associated with more severe reactions include younger age and a shorter duration of AERD [30].

Table 7.1 Standard US protocols for aspirin desensitization

Day	Time	Oral aspirin (2-day protocol)	Intranasal ketorolac and oral aspirin (2-day protocol)	Oral aspirin (1-day protocol #1)	Oral aspirin (1-day protocol #2)	Oral aspirin (1-day protocol #3)
Day 1	8:00 am	20–40 mg	1.26 mg Ketorolac (1 spray)	20.25 mg	41 mg	40 mg
	8:30 am		2.52 mg Ketorolac (2 sprays)			
	9:00 am		5.04 mg Ketorolac (4 sprays)			80 mg
	9:30 am		7.56 mg Ketorolac (6 sprays)	41.5 mg	81 mg	
	10:00 am					160 mg
	10:30 am		60 mg Aspirin			
	11:00 am	40–60 mg		81 mg	161 mg	325 mg
	11:30 am					
	12:00 pm					Desensitization complete
	12:30 pm			162.5 mg	325 mg	
	1:00 pm					
	1:30 pm		Instructions and discharge			
	2:00 pm	60–100 mg		325 mg	Desensitization complete	
	2:30 pm					
	3:00 pm			Desensitization complete		
	3:30 pm					
	4:00 pm					
	4:30 pm					
	5:00 pm	Instructions and discharge				
Day 2	8:00 am	100 mg	150 mg			
	11:00 am	160 mg	325 mg			
	2:00 pm	325 mg	Desensitization complete			
	5:00 pm*	Desensitization complete				

*Discharge times vary and are often significantly later due to extra time needed for treating and recovering from allergic reactions

Once a patient exhibits a clinical reaction to aspirin, this is considered a positive aspirin challenge, and the official diagnosis of AERD is made. After complete resolution of symptoms from a challenge, the patient is considered to have completed desensitization only if the aspirin desensitization protocol is carried out to the 325 mg dose of aspirin. After desensitization is complete, patients are placed on a daily maintenance dose of 325 mg or higher of aspirin daily. The range for the dose of daily aspirin after desensitization is from 325 mg daily to 1300 mg daily. The standard recommendation is for 650 mg two times a day for the first 3–6 months after desensitization. If a patient is doing well on this regimen, the dose can be tapered down to 325 mg two times a day or less frequently to 325 mg daily [49, 62]. It should be noted that some patients on a dose of less than 325 mg twice daily may develop recurrence of nasal congestion [63]. In a study by Rozsasi et al., aspirin maintenance doses of 300 mg daily were compared to 100 mg daily. All patients in the latter group, while no patients in the former group, had a recurrence of nasal polyps and required revision ESS within 1 year of desensitization [64]. Therefore, the maintenance dose of aspirin should be no lower than 325 mg daily. As long as patients are compliant with their minimal daily dose of 325 mg, they also maintain a cross-desensitization to COX-1 inhibitors. If more than 2 days of aspirin maintenance are missed, the recommendation is to repeat desensitization prior to resuming aspirin [65].

If patients benefit from ATAD, the recommendation is to continue with treatment indefinitely [53]. Some patients discontinue ATAD because of GI side effects, bleeding, skin rashes, coronary artery vasospasm, laryngeal symptoms, worsening of asthma, rarely acute pancreatitis, or simply because they find it ineffective [24, 66]. If able to tolerate, patients should trial ATAD for at least 6 months. The most common reason for discontinuation is gastritis. Patients with a history of gastrointestinal ulcers should not initiate aspirin desensitization unless deemed safe by their gastroenterologist. The majority of AERD patients are able to tolerate ATAD without any major complications. In a study of 109 AERD patients on ATAD with a maintenance dose ranging from 325 to 1300 mg daily, Sweis et al. demonstrated that only 0.92% developed a notable gastric ulcer with associated bleed and 0.92% experienced anaphylaxis and 98% of patients had no major complications. Complication rates did not correlate with higher maintenance doses of aspirin [67]. The use of aspirin doses larger than 81 mg daily in pregnancy notably increases the risk of bleeding to the patient and the fetus and may predispose to closure of the ductus arteriosus prematurely [68]. Therefore, aspirin desensitization and/or ATAD is avoided during pregnancy [69]. If a patient has a history of a coagulopathy or is taking an anticoagulant/antiplatelet agent, their hematologist should be consulted prior to initiating aspirin desensitization. If asthma is poorly controlled or the patient is severely symptomatic, aspirin desensitization should be delayed until symptoms are better controlled. Patients with a history of eosinophilic esophagitis should avoid aspirin therapy due to exacerbation of gastrointestinal symptoms [70].

One must keep in mind the concept of silent desensitization. This situation arises in patients with a convincing history of AERD; however, during an oral aspirin challenge, no reaction is noted. In such patients, options include the following: (1)

initiation of a trial of ATAD—and if the patient benefits, then aspirin therapy is continued indefinitely— and (2) rechallenge [71]. If rechallenge is planned, the patient abstains from using NSAIDs for 2 weeks, and antihistamines, LTMAs, cromolyn, and ketotifen are all held for 7 days prior to the rechallenge. Additionally, oral steroids are discontinued or weaned to the lowest possible dose prior to the rechallenge. During the rechallenge, a direct dose of 325 mg is administered. If the patient has a reaction, AERD is confirmed as a diagnosis, and desensitization is completed. If the patient has no reaction, AERD is definitively ruled out [71].

It is important to recognize the emerging role of T2 biologics in the management of patients with AERD. Hayashi et al. performed a non-randomized, noncontrolled study of only 18 patients with AERD who completed 12 months of omalizumab (Xolair) treatment. The number of asthma exacerbations, daily doses of systemic steroids, and all asthma and nasal symptoms were significantly improved. Improvement in symptoms occurred as early as within the first week of treatment to within 3 months of starting treatment [72]. In a study by Tuttle et al., patients with AERD who were treated with mepolizumab (Nucala) for at least 3 months demonstrated improvements in nasal congestion, anosmia, and asthma control. Though this study provides support for a role of IL-5 inhibition in the management of AERD, it was retrospective in nature, and the sample size was only 14 patients [73]. Bachert et al. performed two studies that assessed the efficacy of dupilumab (Dupixent) in patients with uncontrolled CRSwNP. These studies were randomized, double-blind, placebo-controlled. In one study, patients received either subcutaneous dupilumab ($N = 143$) or placebo every 2 weeks for 24 weeks. In the other study, patients received either subcutaneous dupilumab ($N = 150$) or placebo every 2 weeks for 52 weeks, every 2 weeks for 24 weeks then every 4 weeks for the remaining 28 weeks ($N = 145$), or placebo every 2 weeks for 52 weeks. In both studies, dupilumab resulted in significant improvements in nasal polyp scores (NPS), nasal congestion and obstruction scores, and Lund-Mackay scores. These findings were also noted in sub-analyses of patients with self-reported AERD [74]. Thus, dupilumab is now recommended for most difficult to control AERD patients who are not candidates for or have had suboptimal responses to ATAD. In AERD patients with concomitant chronic idiopathic urticaria or those with anaphylaxis preventing the successful use of ATAD, omalizumab should theoretically be an effective option; this has not yet been formally studied.

Topical Medical Therapy

In the 2016 International Consensus Statement on Allergy and Rhinology, high-volume nasal saline irrigations (NSI), defined as >200 mL, are strongly recommended as an adjunct to other medical therapies in the treatment of CRS [75]. This recommendation is based on a grade A level of evidence. Recently, nasal steroid irrigations as compared to topical nasal steroid sprays have been demonstrated to be more efficacious in the treatment of CRS postoperatively. That is, patients experienced improvements in nasal blockage, nasal drainage, Lund-Mackay scores, and modified Lund-Kennedy scores with irrigations [76]. Taken together, the aforementioned findings help guide topical management in patients with AERD postoperatively. For AERD patients, topical treatment should be high-volume nasal irrigations with dissolved steroids rather than topical steroid sprays. Options for dissolved steroids include 0.5 mg budesonide or 1–2 mg mometasone in 240 mL of isotonic saline. Rinses should be performed twice daily (approximately 120 mL per nostril with each rinse). Furthermore, with the steroid being dissolved in 240 mL of saline, studies show that the total concentration of steroid retained in the sinuses is equivalent between steroid sprays and steroid irrigations [76]. Another potential option is the exhalation delivery system (EDS), that is, EDS with fluticasone (EDS-FLU). This delivery system has been shown, as compared to conventional topical steroid sprays, to penetrate deeper and higher in to the nasal cavities and paranasal sinuses [77, 78]. Like nasal steroid irrigations, we would recommend EDS-FLU over topical steroid sprays in AERD patients. EDS-FLU, however, is FDA approved in adults with CRSwNP, while steroid irrigations are not. EDS-FLU may also be a good alternative for AERD patients who cannot tolerate irrigations.

As detailed above, aspirin desensitization and ATAD in the United States are carried out using oral aspirin. In Europe, aspirin desensitization and ATAD can be conducted with intranasal lysine aspirin. Howe et al. demonstrated that treatment resulted in improved quality of life in 60 of 78 patients at 3 months post-desensitization and 19 of 27 patients at 12 months post-desensitization. Moreover, there was a significant decrease in emergency visits, oral steroid use, and hospitalizations in those on nasal lysine aspirin for a year. One other advantage in this study was overall lower gastrointestinal side effects in AERD patients treated with nasal lysine aspirin as compared to those treated with oral aspirin, that is, 14% versus 3.8% [62, 79]. However, cross-desensitization with oral aspirin and other COX-1-inhibiting NSAIDs would not be expected to occur with topical lysine aspirin therapy.

In patients with AERD, an appropriate technique for the delivery of topical medications to both the upper and lower airways is critical. Thomas et al. demonstrated the head-down-and-forward position is most efficacious for the delivery of nasal irrigations to the sinuses [80]. With regard to asthma control, numerous studies have demonstrated 76% compliance with the use of inhaled corticosteroids but only 46% performing proper technique. In patients with AERD, counseling on technique is important to long-term management [81].

In AERD patients, asthma should be optimally controlled and aggressively targeted per the Global Initiative for Asthma (GINA) 2019 guidelines [82]. Topical treatments are preferred as first-line agents to control asthma. Per these guidelines, the most commonly used treatments include inhaled corticosteroids (ICS) and long-acting beta-agonists (LABAs). In AERD patients, CRSwNP should be optimally controlled with intranasal corticosteroids. As in all patients, topical alpha-adrenergic decongestants are not recommended long-term due to the risk of development of rhinitis medicamentosa [83].

Overview of Evidence Supporting Medical Therapy (or Lack Thereof)

We have reviewed the various medical therapies (i.e., corticosteroids, LTMAs, ATAD, T2 biologics, topical delivery mechanisms) and the specific evidence for their respective roles in the treatment of AERD. Fortunately, systemic corticosteroids, once the mainstay of AERD medical therapy, are being replaced by ATAD, LTMAs, and T2 biological therapies. The most robust data and the longest studied therapy is ATAD which appears to be most effective following a complete ESS. ATAD has been shown to maintain SNOT-22 improvements post-ESS in two studies. In addition, there are improved smell scores, reduced oral corticosteroid usage, fewer antibiotic prescriptions, and improved tolerance to alcohol [84, 85]. LTMAs also play a role in medical therapy, with studies suggesting zileuton to be superior to CysLT1 antagonists like montelukast, providing both upper (rhinorrhea, olfaction, and nasal congestion) and lower airway (FEV1) benefit [31]. Finally, early emerging data suggests that T2 biologics may be effective medical therapy for AERD. More data specifically studying the AERD subset of CRSwNP will likely be forthcoming. In AERD patients who are responders to ATAD, there has been a resultant improvement in both upper and lower airway symptoms and a decrease in the number of revision surgeries needed [86]. All the while, the quality of life of AERD patients is notably improved. Additionally, ATAD has been demonstrated to be economically cost-effective [87]. This finding is important when patients are considering other medical therapies, that is, T2 biological therapy. The average annual cost for T2 biological therapy ranges from $31,000 to $39,000 per patient [88]. ASA desensitization is now more widely available than ever before and has shown to be cost-effective. Aspirin itself is quite inexpensive. Therefore, ATAD following complete ESS should be considered the mainstay of treatment for most AERD patients that do not respond to topical corticosteroid and LTMA therapy, unless contraindicated. With regard to topical therapies, high-volume low-pressure, high-volume high-pressure, and/or exhalation delivery systems are the preferred choice of topical medication delivery in AERD patients.

Surgical Management and Outcomes

Surgical Approach

In patients with CRS and comorbid asthma, ESS has been shown to improve upper and lower airway symptoms as well as decrease the total dosage and total number of days of systemic steroids needed by patients for management of their asthma postoperatively [89]. Therefore, ESS is a critical part of the overall treatment algorithm for AERD. AERD, though a challenging disease process that requires multi-modality treatment, has been shown to respond positively on multiple levels following ESS. There is no question that patients with AERD have an extensive inflammatory polypoid burden. One would expect that patients with AERD who undergo ESS would have better outcomes with complete ESS as compared to targeted ESS. Not only is more disease burden removed in complete ESS, but also more efficacious delivery of long-term postoperative topical delivery of medications should be accomplished. The literature makes it clear that topical long-term treatment is critical to improved outcomes after ESS [90]. Complete ESS includes bilateral frontal sinusotomy, anterior and posterior ethmoidectomy, maxillary antrostomy, and sphenoidotomy. Targeted ESS is any surgical intervention that does not fulfill the criteria of complete ESS. To provide clarity on this issue, Deconde et al. performed a prospective analysis comparing quality-of-life outcomes in patients undergoing complete versus targeted ESS. Three hundred and eleven patients were enrolled in the study, and there was a statistically significant improvement in SNOT-22 scores in the complete ESS group when compared to the targeted ESS group ($p = 0.011$). Also, in this cohort of patients, there was a statistically significantly higher number of AERD patients in the group that underwent complete ESS ($p = 0.002$) [91]. In a retrospective analysis, Adappa et al. shed light on a different advantage of complete ESS in patients with AERD. In their study, 32 patients underwent complete ESS followed by aspirin desensitization and ATAD. Patients were followed for 30 months and demonstrated stably improved quality-of-life scores, concluding that complete ESS followed by timely aspirin desensitization and maintenance therapy is an effective combination in the long-term management of AERD patients [84]. Other studies have focused on the timing of desensitization, when it is optimal. Jerschow et al. completed a prospective study in which patients completed aspirin desensitization either before ESS or 3–4 weeks after ESS. The upper and lower airway reactions during desensitization were unanimously decreased in the group that underwent aspirin desensitization after ESS [86]. Additionally, undergoing ESS prior to aspirin desensitization obviates the need for aspirin cessation and bleeding risk in the perioperative period.

The literature has also investigated the role of extended frontal sinus surgery, including Draf IIA, IIB, or III (endoscopic modified Lothrop), in AERD patients. Barham et al. completed a cadaveric study that demonstrated Draf III was superior to Draf IIa for facilitating topical irrigations, particularly when in vertex head position [92]. It is important to recognize that Draf III can be indicated in patients with the refractory disease despite prior ESS or as a primary procedure in those with severe polyposis and specific comorbidities such as AERD, asthma, or ciliary dyskinesia [93]. Various studies have analyzed long-term outcomes of Draf III in nasal polyposis patients. One retrospective study of 338 CRSwNP patients (62 of which had AERD) demonstrated that polyp recurrence was 36% 12 months after Draf III as compared to 49% in Draf IIa frontal sinusotomy [94]. Other studies have identified risk factors for frontal sinus restenosis and the need for revision frontal sinus surgery. These risk factors include intraoperative frontal ostium size as well as the presence of eosinophilic inflammation. One such study was by Ting et al., which retrospectively reported in 204 patients a 30% revision rate following Draf III frontal sinusotomy [95]. Naidoo et al. reported a retrospective study in which only 5% of their 229 Draf III patients required revision surgery at a 45-month follow-up [96]. Another retrospective study reported only a 12% revision Draf III rate [97].

Draf III can be completed in the traditional "inside-out" technique, in which the aforementioned studies were completed. A variation to the Draf III technique is termed "outside-in". Wong et al. reported on this technique in a case series of 104 patients, 13 of whom had AERD. The results demonstrated that patients as a whole had improvements in quality-of-life scores following the "outside-in" technique, but the 13 AERD patients experienced overall poorer clinical outcomes comparatively [98]. Regardless of the Draf III technique utilized, there exists enough evidence to support the early use of Draf III as part of a complete ESS in the management of AERD. Yet unpublished data from the University of Pennsylvania further supports this surgical approach. In this study, a large cohort of AERD patients who underwent Draf III and aspirin desensitization following surgery had improved SNOT-22 scores which were sustained at greater than 30 months of follow-up, with surgical revision rate of less than 5%.

With advancements in instrumentation, Draf III can be completed more efficiently and safely for patients. Despite the aforementioned benefits and such advancements, Draf III is not without morbidities. Patients should be clearly counseled on the associated risks. Patel et al. compared complications between Draf IIB and Draf III. Neither group had major complications (CSF leak, posterior table injury, visual compromise, anosmia, tension pneumocephalus, or meningitis). The Draf III cohort had an 11.8% minor complication rate, and the Draf IIB cohort had a 14.3% minor complication rate ($p = 1.0$). Minor complications included hyposmia, prolonged crusting, adhesions, epistaxis, and nasal bone dehiscence [99].

Overview of Evidence Supporting Surgical Therapy (or Lack Thereof)

AERD is a difficult disease process to treat, but surgical intervention is essential in almost all cases to achieving symptomatic improvement. Complete ESS is preferred over targeted ESS, and in complete ESS, there is support in the literature for the use of Draf III during primary surgery rather than a salvage option. This surgical approach will ultimately allow for overall decreased disease burden and efficacious delivery of long-term topical treatment. By diminishing the overall disease burden, ESS should precede aspirin desensitization and has been shown to improve long-term outcomes for patients on ATAD. In patients with AERD, the benefits of a Draf III frontal sinusotomy outweigh the morbidity with which it is associated.

Impact of Rhinologic Interventions on Medical Disorder

The combination of complete ESS and aspirin desensitization with ATAD results in improved subjective and objective outcome measures. Several studies demonstrate a statistically significant improvement in SNOT-20 and SNOT-22 scores 4 weeks following ESS. Moreover, such studies go on to demonstrate stably improved symptoms after aspirin desensitization while on ATAD for up to 30 months after ESS [84, 100, 101]. In addition, there are improved smell scores, decreased use of oral corticosteroid and antibiotic prescriptions, and patients report improved tolerance to alcohol. Nasal polyp recurrence and revision ESS rates were significantly lower in patients maintained on ATAD when compared to those who only completed ESS [54, 84, 101]. ESS decreases overall disease burden in AERD patients and improves tolerability and responsiveness to aspirin desensitization and ATAD, particularly in patients who failed desensitization in the past [85, 102]. Regarding the extent of a complete ESS, Draf III has been shown in various studies to improve the delivery of postoperative topical therapies while minimizing the revision ESS rates. Therefore, in patients with AERD, there should be a low threshold to perform a Draf III. High-quality randomized control trials are still needed to further delineate the optimal extent of surgery.

Case Presentation

A 35-year-old man experienced an evolving set of upper and lower airway symptoms. Symptoms were preceded by an intractable upper respiratory tract infection in his late 20s. Within a year of this infection, he developed an abrupt onset of asthma. A few years later, he was noted to have diffuse and widespread nasal polyps for which he underwent endoscopic sinus surgery. His diffuse nasal polyposis recurred within 6 months of surgery, and he was noted to have a de novo allergy to NSAIDs that resulted in a brief hospitalization for acute respiratory distress. At this point, the patient's medications include prednisone 10 mg daily, amoxicillin-clavulanate 875/125 mg twice daily, fluticasone-salmeterol 250/50 mg one puff twice daily, and montelukast 10 mg daily. He was referred to the division of rhinology at a tertiary care center for further workup and management.

Management and Outcomes

On presentation, a thorough history was obtained. Physical exam was completed, including nasal endoscopy. Diffuse nasal polyposis was noted bilaterally. An interval CT sinus was obtained and demonstrated bilateral complete opacification. The physical exam findings coupled with the patient's history as noted in the vignette were suggestive of AERD. He was referred to our AERD center. Given the convincing history of AERD, the patient was scheduled for revision ESS to diminish his polyp burden. The extent of surgery included bilateral maxillary antrostomies, bilateral total ethmoidectomies, bilateral sphenoidotomies, and Draf III frontal sinusotomy. One month preoperatively, the patient underwent an aspirin challenge, which confirmed his diagnosis of AERD. Six weeks postoperatively, he completed a two-day aspirin desensitization procedure.

Per the hybrid Intranasal ketorolac/modified aspirin protocol, the patient received intranasal ketorolac at a low dose, with a gradual progression to higher doses. The patient then switched to oral aspirin at low, then medium, and then full doses. During desensitization, the patient was treated for any asthmatic or nasal reactions and was monitored until he was fully recovered. The dose to which the patient reacted was repeated and tolerated before increasing further. Ultimately, the patient reached a dose of 325 mg of aspirin at the end of day two of the desensitization protocol. This completed his desensitization.

Six months after desensitization, the patient continues to take 325 mg aspirin twice daily. He has not experienced a recurrence of his nasal polyps or respiratory symptoms. Nasal endoscopy and CT sinus 6 months postoperatively clearly demonstrate these improved findings. Additionally, the patient substantially reduced his dependence on oral steroids and antibiotics.

Conclusion

AERD is associated with disturbances in arachidonic acid metabolism, resulting in an imbalance of inflammatory mediators. In effect, patients experience upper and lower airway inflammation manifesting as CRSwNP and asthma. Though the clinical presentation may lead one to the diagnosis, definitive diagnosis of AERD requires an aspirin challenge. Treatment requires multi-modality therapy. For long-term management of AERD and to minimize the use of systemic corticosteroids, we recommend complete ESS followed by aspirin desensitization and ATAD. Adjunctive treatments include LTMAs and topical steroids. T2 biologics should be reserved for AERD patients who cannot tolerate or do not respond favorably to aspirin desensitization and/or ATAD.

References

1. Cardet JC, White AA, Barrett NA, Feldweg AM, Wickner PG, Savage J, et al. Alcohol-induced respiratory symptoms are common in patients with aspirin exacerbated respiratory disease. J Allergy Clin Immunol Pract. 2014;2(2):208–13.
2. Berges-Gimeno MP, Simon RA, Stevenson DD. The natural history and clinical characteristics of aspirin-exacerbated respiratory disease. Ann Allergy Asthma Immunol. 2002;89(5):474–8.
3. Szczeklik A, Nizankowska E, Duplaga M. Natural history of aspirin-induced asthma. AIANE Investigators. European Network on Aspirin-Induced Asthma. Eur Respir J. 2000;16(3):432–6.
4. Tajudeen BA, Schwartz JS, Bosso JV. The role of aspirin desensitization in the management of aspirin-exacerbated respiratory disease. Curr Opin Otolaryngol Head Neck Surg. 2017;25(1):30–4.
5. Rajan JP, Wineinger NE, Stevenson DD, White AA. Prevalence of aspirin-exacerbated respiratory disease among asthmatic patients: a meta-analysis of the literature. J Allergy Clin Immunol. 2015;135(3):676–81.e1.

6. Stevens WW, Peters AT, Hirsch AG, Nordberg CM, Schwartz BS, Mercer DG, et al. Clinical characteristics of patients with chronic rhinosinusitis with nasal polyps, asthma, and aspirin-exacerbated respiratory disease. J Allergy Clin Immunol Pract. 2017;5(4):1061–1070.e3.
7. Cahill KN, Johns CB, Cui J, Wickner P, Bates DW, Laidlaw TM, et al. Automated identification of an aspirin-exacerbated respiratory disease cohort. J Allergy Clin Immunol. 2017;139(3):819–825.e6.
8. Buchheit K, Bensko J, Lewis E, Gakpo D, Laidlaw T. The importance of timely diagnosis of aspirin-exacerbated respiratory disease for patient health and safety [Manuscript in Preparation].
9. White AA, Stevenson DD. Aspirin-exacerbated respiratory disease. N Engl J Med. 2018;379(23):2281–2.
10. Christie PE, Tagari P, Ford-Hutchinson AW, Charlesson S, Chee P, Arm JP, et al. Urinary leukotriene E4 concentrations increase after aspirin challenge in aspirin-sensitive asthmatic subjects. Am Rev Respir Dis. 1991;143(5 Pt 1):1025–9.
11. Bosso JV, Schwartz LB, Stevenson DD. Tryptase and histamine release during aspirin-induced respiratory reactions. J Allergy Clin Immunol. 1991;88(6):830–7.
12. Wells E, Jackson CG, Harper ST, Mann J, Eady RP. Characterization of primate bronchoalveolar mast cells. II. Inhibition of histamine, LTC4, and PGD2 release from primate bronchoalveolar mast cells and a comparison with rat peritoneal mast cells. J Immunol. 1986;137(12):3941–5.
13. Robuschi M, Gambaro G, Sestini P, Pieroni MG, Refini RM, Vaghi A, et al. Attenuation of aspirin-induced bronchoconstriction by sodium cromoglycate and nedocromil sodium. Am J Respir Crit Care Med. 1997;155(4):1461–4.
14. Cowburn AS, Sladek K, Soja J, Adamek L, Nizankowska E, Szczeklik A, et al. Overexpression of leukotriene C4 synthase in bronchial biopsies from patients with aspirin-intolerant asthma. J Clin Invest. 1998;101(4):834–46.
15. Laidlaw TM, Kidder MS, Bhattacharyya N, Xing W, Shen S, Milne GL, et al. Cysteinyl leukotriene overproduction in aspirin-exacerbated respiratory disease is driven by platelet-adherent leukocytes. Blood. 2012;119(16):3790–8.
16. Liu T, Laidlaw TM, Katz HR, Boyce JA. Prostaglandin E2 deficiency causes a phenotype of aspirin sensitivity that depends on platelets and cysteinyl leukotrienes. Proc Natl Acad Sci U S A. 2013;110(42):16987–92.
17. Uematsu S, Matsumoto M, Takeda K, Akira S. Lipopolysaccharide-dependent prostaglandin E(2) production is regulated by the glutathione-dependent prostaglandin E(2) synthase gene induced by the Toll-like receptor 4/MyD88/NF-IL6 pathway. J Immunol. 2002;168(11):5811–6.
18. Roca-Ferrer J, Garcia-Garcia FJ, Pereda J, Perez-Gonzalez M, Pujols L, Alobid I, et al. Reduced expression of COXs and production of prostaglandin E(2) in patients with nasal polyps with or without aspirin-intolerant asthma. J Allergy Clin Immunol. 2011;128(1):66–72.e1.
19. Kay LJ, Yeo WW, Peachell PT. Prostaglandin E2 activates EP2 receptors to inhibit human lung mast cell degranulation. Br J Pharmacol. 2006;147(7):707–13.
20. Säfholm J, Manson ML, Bood J, Delin I, Orre AC, Bergman P, et al. Prostaglandin E2 inhibits mast cell-dependent bronchoconstriction in human small airways through the E prostanoid subtype 2 receptor. J Allergy Clin Immunol. 2015;136(5):1232–9.e1.
21. Flamand N, Surette ME, Picard S, Bourgoin S, Borgeat P. Cyclic AMP-mediated inhibition of 5-lipoxygenase translocation and leukotriene biosynthesis in human neutrophils. Mol Pharmacol. 2002;62(2):250–6.
22. Petrucci G, De Cristofaro R, Rutella S, Ranelletti FO, Pocaterra D, Lancellotti S, et al. Prostaglandin E2 differentially modulates human platelet function through the prostanoid EP2 and EP3 receptors. J Pharmacol Exp Ther. 2011;336(2):391–402.
23. Ying S, Meng Q, Scadding G, Parikh A, Corrigan CJ, Lee TH. Aspirin-sensitive rhinosinusitis is associated with reduced E-prostanoid 2 receptor expression on nasal mucosal inflammatory cells. J Allergy Clin Immunol. 2006;117(2):312–8.

24. Cahill KN, Raby BA, Zhou X, Guo F, Thibault D, Baccarelli A, et al. Impaired E Prostanoid2 expression and resistance to prostaglandin E2 in nasal polyp fibroblasts from subjects with aspirin-exacerbated respiratory disease. Am J Respir Cell Mol Biol. 2016;54(1):34–40.
25. Chang JE, Ding D, Martin-Lazaro J, White A, Stevenson DD. Smoking, environmental tobacco smoke, and aspirin-exacerbated respiratory disease. Ann Allergy Asthma Immunol. 2012;108(1):14–9.
26. Van Sambeek R, Stevenson DD, Baldasaro M, Lam BK, Zhao J, Yoshida S, et al. 5′ flanking region polymorphism of the gene encoding leukotriene C4 synthase does not correlate with the aspirin-intolerant asthma phenotype in the United States. J Allergy Clin Immunol. 2000;106(1 Pt 1):72–6.
27. Jerschow E, Edin ML, Pelletier T, Abuzeid WM, Akbar NA, Gibber M, et al. Plasma 15-hydroxyeicosatetraenoic acid predicts treatment outcomes in aspirin-exacerbated respiratory disease. J Allergy Clin Immunol Pract. 2017;5(4):998–1007.e2.
28. Fan Y, Feng S, Xia W, Qu L, Li X, Chen S, et al. Aspirin-exacerbated respiratory disease in China: a cohort investigation and literature review. Am J Rhinol Allergy. 2012;26(1):e20–2.
29. Fahrenholz JM. Natural history and clinical features of aspirin-exacerbated respiratory disease. Clin Rev Allergy Immunol. 2003;24(2):113–24.
30. Hope AP, Woessner KA, Simon RA, Stevenson DD. Rational approach to aspirin dosing during oral challenges and desensitization of patients with aspirin-exacerbated respiratory disease. J Allergy Clin Immunol. 2009;123(2):406–10.
31. Ta V, White AA. Survey-defined patient experiences with aspirin-exacerbated respiratory disease. J Allergy Clin Immunol Pract. 2015;3(5):711–8.
32. Jenkins C, Costello J, Hodge L. Systematic review of prevalence of aspirin induced asthma and its implications for clinical practice. BMJ. 2004;328(7437):434.
33. Szczeklik A, Stevenson DD. Aspirin-induced asthma: advances in pathogenesis, diagnosis, and management. J Allergy Clin Immunol. 2003;111(5):913–21; quiz 922
34. Cahill KN, Bensko JC, Boyce JA, Laidlaw TM. Prostaglandin D_2: a dominant mediator of aspirin-exacerbated respiratory disease. J Allergy Clin Immunol. 2015;135(1):245–52.
35. Shah NH, Schneider TR, DeFaria YD, Cahill KN, Laidlaw TM. Eosinophilia-associated coronary artery vasospasm in patients with aspirin-exacerbated respiratory disease. J Allergy Clin Immunol Pract. 2016;4(6):1215–9.
36. Lee-Sarwar K, Johns C, Laidlaw TM, Cahill KN. Tolerance of daily low-dose aspirin does not preclude aspirin-exacerbated respiratory disease. J Allergy Clin Immunol Pract. 2015;3(3):449–51.
37. Israel E, Fischer AR, Rosenberg MA, Lilly CM, Callery JC, Shapiro J, et al. The pivotal role of 5-lipoxygenase products in the reaction of aspirin-sensitive asthmatics to aspirin. Am Rev Respir Dis. 1993;148(6 Pt 1):1447–51.
38. Stevenson DD, Simon RA, Mathison DA, Christiansen SC. Montelukast is only partially effective in inhibiting aspirin responses in aspirin-sensitive asthmatics. Ann Allergy Asthma Immunol. 2000;85(6 Pt 1):477–82.
39. Dursun AB, Woessner KA, Simon RA, Karasoy D, Stevenson DD. Predicting outcomes of oral aspirin challenges in patients with asthma, nasal polyps, and chronic sinusitis. Ann Allergy Asthma Immunol. 2008;100(5):420–5.
40. Celejewska-Wójcik N, Mastalerz L, Wójcik K, Nieckarz R, Januszek R, Hartwich P, et al. Incidence of aspirin hypersensitivity in patients with chronic rhinosinusitis and diagnostic value of urinary leukotriene E4. Pol Arch Med Wewn. 2012;122(9):422–7.
41. Divekar R, Hagan J, Rank M, Park M, Volcheck G, O'Brien E, et al. Diagnostic utility of urinary LTE4 in asthma, allergic rhinitis, chronic rhinosinusitis, nasal polyps, and aspirin sensitivity. J Allergy Clin Immunol Pract. 2016;4(4):665–70.
42. Mascia K, Borish L, Patrie J, Hunt J, Phillips CD, Steinke JW. Chronic hyperplastic eosinophilic sinusitis as a predictor of aspirin-exacerbated respiratory disease. Ann Allergy Asthma Immunol. 2005;94(6):652–7.

43. Lin DC, Chandra RK, Tan BK, Zirkle W, Conley DB, Grammer LC, et al. Association between severity of asthma and degree of chronic rhinosinusitis. Am J Rhinol Allergy. 2011;25(4):205–8.
44. Alobid I, Benitez P, Pujols L, Maldonado M, Bernal-Sprekelsen M, Morello A, et al. Severe nasal polyposis and its impact on quality of life. The effect of a short course of oral steroids followed by long-term intranasal steroid treatment. Rhinology. 2006;44(1):8–13.
45. Suh YJ, Yoon SH, Sampson AP, Kim HJ, Kim SH, Nahm DH, et al. Specific immunoglobulin E for staphylococcal enterotoxins in nasal polyps from patients with aspirin-intolerant asthma. Clin Exp Allergy. 2004;34(8):1270–5.
46. Fokkens WJ, Lund VJ, Mullol J, Bachert C, Alobid I, Baroody F, et al. EPOS 2012: European position paper on rhinosinusitis and nasal polyps 2012. A summary for otorhinolaryngologists. Rhinology. 2012;50(1):1–12.
47. Dahlén SE, Malmström K, Nizankowska E, Dahlén B, Kuna P, Kowalski M, et al. Improvement of aspirin-intolerant asthma by montelukast, a leukotriene antagonist: a randomized, double-blind, placebo-controlled trial. Am J Respir Crit Care Med. 2002;165(1):9–14.
48. Dahlén B, Nizankowska E, Szczeklik A, Zetterström O, Bochenek G, Kumlin M, et al. Benefits from adding the 5-lipoxygenase inhibitor zileuton to conventional therapy in aspirin-intolerant asthmatics. Am J Respir Crit Care Med. 1998;157(4 Pt 1):1187–94.
49. Lee JY, Simon RA, Stevenson DD. Selection of aspirin dosages for aspirin desensitization treatment in patients with aspirin-exacerbated respiratory disease. J Allergy Clin Immunol. 2007;119(1):157–64.
50. Laidlaw TM, Fuentes DJ, Wang Y. Efficacy of zileuton in patients with asthma and history of aspirin sensitivity: a retrospective analysis of data from two phase 3 studies. J Allergy Clin Immunol. 2017;139(2):AB384.
51. Morales DR, Lipworth BJ, Guthrie B, Jackson C, Donnan PT, Santiago VH. Safety risks for patients with aspirin-exacerbated respiratory disease after acute exposure to selective non-steroidal anti-inflammatory drugs and COX-2 inhibitors: meta-analysis of controlled clinical trials. J Allergy Clin Immunol. 2014;134(1):40–5.
52. Settipane RA, Stevenson DD. Cross sensitivity with acetaminophen in aspirin-sensitive subjects with asthma. J Allergy Clin Immunol. 1989;84(1):26–33.
53. Walters KM, Waldram JD, Woessner KM, White AA. Long-term clinical outcomes of aspirin desensitization with continuous daily aspirin therapy in aspirin-exacerbated respiratory disease. Am J Rhinol Allergy. 2018;32(4):280–6.
54. Levy JM, Rudmik L, Peters AT, Wise SK, Rotenberg BW, Smith TL. Contemporary management of chronic rhinosinusitis with nasal polyposis in aspirin-exacerbated respiratory disease: an evidence-based review with recommendations. Int Forum Allergy Rhinol. 2016;6(12):1273–83.
55. Stewart RA, Ram B, Hamilton G, Weiner J, Kane KJ. Montelukast as an adjunct to oral and inhaled steroid therapy in chronic nasal polyposis. Otolaryngol Head Neck Surg. 2008;139(5):682–7.
56. White AA, Stevenson DD, Simon RA. The blocking effect of essential controller medications during aspirin challenges in patients with aspirin-exacerbated respiratory disease. Ann Allergy Asthma Immunol. 2005;95(4):330–5.
57. Szczeklik A, Serwonska M. Inhibition of idiosyncratic reactions to aspirin in asthmatic patients by clemastine. Thorax. 1979;34(5):654–7.
58. DeGregorio GA, Singer J, Cahill KN, Laidlaw T. A 1-day, 90-minute aspirin challenge and desensitization protocol in aspirin-exacerbated respiratory disease. J Allergy Clin Immunol Pract. 2019;7(4):1174–80.
59. Waldram J, Walters K, Simon R, Woessner K, Waalen J, White A. Safety and outcomes of aspirin desensitization for aspirin-exacerbated respiratory disease: a single-center study. J Allergy Clin Immunol. 2018;141(1):250–6.
60. Lee RU, White AA, Ding D, Dursun AB, Woessner KM, Simon RA, et al. Use of intranasal ketorolac and modified oral aspirin challenge for desensitization of aspirin-exacerbated respiratory disease. Ann Allergy Asthma Immunol. 2010;105(2):130–5.

61. White A, Ludington E, Mehra P, Stevenson DD, Simon RA. Effect of leukotriene modifier drugs on the safety of oral aspirin challenges. Ann Allergy Asthma Immunol. 2006;97(5):688–93.

62. Berges-Gimeno MP, Simon RA, Stevenson DD. Long-term treatment with aspirin desensitization in asthmatic patients with aspirin-exacerbated respiratory disease. J Allergy Clin Immunol. 2003;111(1):180–6.

63. Stevenson DD, Pleskow WW, Simon RA, Mathison DA, Lumry WR, Schatz M, et al. Aspirin-sensitive rhinosinusitis asthma: a double-blind crossover study of treatment with aspirin. J Allergy Clin Immunol. 1984;73(4):500–7.

64. Rozsasi A, Polzehl D, Deutschle T, Smith E, Wiesmiller K, Riechelmann H, et al. Long-term treatment with aspirin desensitization: a prospective clinical trial comparing 100 and 300 mg aspirin daily. Allergy. 2008;63(9):1228–34.

65. Pleskow WW, Stevenson DD, Mathison DA, Simon RA, Schatz M, Zeiger RS. Aspirin desensitization in aspirin-sensitive asthmatic patients: clinical manifestations and characterization of the refractory period. J Allergy Clin Immunol. 1982;69(1 Pt 1):11–9.

66. Durrani SR, Kelly JT. Pancreatitis as a complication of aspirin desensitization for aspirin-exacerbated respiratory disease. J Allergy Clin Immunol. 2013;131(1):244–6.

67. Sweis A, Lock T, Ig-Izevbekhai K, Lin T, Gleeson P, Civantos A, et al. Major Complications of Aspirin Desensitization and Maintenance Therapy in Aspirin Exacerbated Respiratory Disease. Int Forum Allergy Rhinol. 2020. https://doi.org/10.1002/alr.22643. In Press.

68. Hertz-Picciotto I, Hopenhayn-Rich C, Golub M, Hooper K. The risks and benefits of taking aspirin during pregnancy. Epidemiol Rev. 1990;12:108–48.

69. James AH, Brancazio LR, Price T. Aspirin and reproductive outcomes. Obstet Gynecol Surv. 2008;63(1):49–57.

70. Eid RC, Palumbo ML, Laidlaw TM, Buchheit KM, Cahill KN. A retrospective analysis of esophageal eosinophilia in patients with aspirin-exacerbated respiratory disease. J Allergy Clin Immunol Pract. 2019;7(4):1338–40.

71. White AA, Bosso JV, Stevenson DD. The clinical dilemma of "silent desensitization" in aspirin-exacerbated respiratory disease. Allergy Asthma Proc. 2013;34(4):378–82.

72. Hayashi H, Mitsui C, Nakatani E, Fukutomi Y, Kajiwara K, Watai K, et al. Omalizumab reduces cysteinyl leukotriene and $9\alpha,11\beta$-prostaglandin F2 overproduction in aspirin-exacerbated respiratory disease. J Allergy Clin Immunol. 2016;137(5):1585–1587.e4.

73. Tuttle KL, Buchheit KM, Laidlaw TM, Cahill KN. A retrospective analysis of mepolizumab in subjects with aspirin-exacerbated respiratory disease. J Allergy Clin Immunol Pract. 2018;6(3):1045–7.

74. Bachert C, Han JK, Desrosiers M, Hellings PW, Amin N, Lee SE, et al. Efficacy and safety of dupilumab in patients with severe chronic rhinosinusitis with nasal polyps (LIBERTY NP SINUS-24 and LIBERTY NP SINUS-52): results from two multicentre, randomised, double-blind, placebo-controlled, parallel-group phase 3 trials. Lancet. 2019;394(10209):1638–50.

75. Orlandi RR, Kingdom TT, Hwang PH. International consensus statement on allergy and rhinology: rhinosinusitis executive summary. Int Forum Allergy Rhinol. 2016;6(Suppl 1):S3–21.

76. Harvey RJ, Snidvongs K, Kalish LH, Oakley GM, Sacks R. Corticosteroid nasal irrigations are more effective than simple sprays in a randomized double-blinded placebo-controlled trial for chronic rhinosinusitis after sinus surgery. Int Forum Allergy Rhinol. 2018;8(4):461–70.

77. Leopold DA, Elkayam D, Messina JC, Kosik-Gonzalez C, Djupesland PG, Mahmoud RA. NAVIGATE II: randomized, double-blind trial of the exhalation delivery system with fluticasone for nasal polyposis. J Allergy Clin Immunol. 2019;143(1):126–134.e5.

78. Sindwani R, Han JK, Soteres DF, Messina JC, Carothers JL, Mahmoud RA, et al. NAVIGATE I: randomized, placebo-controlled, double-blind trial of the exhalation delivery system with fluticasone for chronic rhinosinusitis with nasal polyps. Am J Rhinol Allergy. 2019;33(1):69–82.

79. Howe R, Mirakian RM, Pillai P, Gane S, Darby YC, Scadding GK. Audit of nasal lysine aspirin therapy in recalcitrant aspirin exacerbated respiratory disease. World Allergy Organ J. 2014;7(1):18.

80. Thomas WW, Harvey RJ, Rudmik L, Hwang PH, Schlosser RJ. Distribution of topical agents to the paranasal sinuses: an evidence-based review with recommendations. Int Forum Allergy Rhinol. 2013;3(9):691–703.
81. Cochrane MG, Bala MV, Downs KE, Mauskopf J, Ben-Joseph RH. Inhaled corticosteroids for asthma therapy: patient compliance, devices, and inhalation technique. Chest. 2000;117(2):542–50.
82. 2019 GINA Main Report – Global Initiative for Asthma – GINA [Internet]. Global Initiative for Asthma – GINA. 2020 [Cited 1 Feb 2020]. Available from: https://ginasthma.org/gina-reports
83. Mortuaire G, de Gabory L, François M, Massé G, Bloch F, Brion N, et al. Rebound congestion and rhinitis medicamentosa: nasal decongestants in clinical practice. Critical review of the literature by a medical panel. Eur Ann Otorhinolaryngol Head Neck Dis. 2013;130(3):137–44.
84. Adappa ND, Ranasinghe VJ, Trope M, Brooks SG, Glicksman JT, Parasher AK, et al. Outcomes after complete endoscopic sinus surgery and aspirin desensitization in aspirin-exacerbated respiratory disease. Int Forum Allergy Rhinol. 2018;8(1):49–53.
85. Shah SJ, Abuzeid WM, Ponduri A, Pelletier T, Ren Z, Keskin T, et al. Endoscopic sinus surgery improves aspirin treatment response in aspirin-exacerbated respiratory disease patients. Int Forum Allergy Rhinol. 2019;9(12):1401–8.
86. Jerschow E, Edin ML, Chi Y, Hurst B, Abuzeid WM, Akbar NA, et al. Sinus surgery is associated with a decrease in aspirin-induced reaction severity in patients with aspirin exacerbated respiratory disease. J Allergy Clin Immunol Pract. 2019;7(5):1580–8.
87. Shaker M, Lobb A, Jenkins P, O'Rourke D, Takemoto SK, Sheth S, et al. An economic analysis of aspirin desensitization in aspirin-exacerbated respiratory disease. J Allergy Clin Immunol. 2008;121(1):81–7.
88. Anderson WC, Szefler SJ. Cost-effectiveness and comparative effectiveness of biologic therapy for asthma: to biologic or not to biologic. Ann Allergy Asthma Immunol. 2019;122(4):367–72.
89. Palmer JN, Conley DB, Dong RG, Ditto AM, Yarnold PR, Kern RC. Efficacy of endoscopic sinus surgery in the management of patients with asthma and chronic sinusitis. Am J Rhinol. 2001;15(1):49–53.
90. Rudmik L, Soler ZM, Orlandi RR, Stewart MG, Bhattacharyya N, Kennedy DW, et al. Early postoperative care following endoscopic sinus surgery: an evidence-based review with recommendations. Int Forum Allergy Rhinol. 2011;1(6):417–30.
91. DeConde AS, Suh JD, Mace JC, Alt JA, Smith TL. Outcomes of complete vs targeted approaches to endoscopic sinus surgery. Int Forum Allergy Rhinol. 2015;5(8):691–700.
92. Barham HP, Ramakrishnan VR, Knisely A, Do TQ, Chan LS, Gunaratne DA, et al. Frontal sinus surgery and sinus distribution of nasal irrigation. Int Forum Allergy Rhinol. 2016;6(3):238–42.
93. Orgain CA, Harvey RJ. The role of frontal sinus drillouts in nasal polyposis. Curr Opin Otolaryngol Head Neck Surg. 2018;26(1):34–40.
94. Bassiouni A, Wormald PJ. Role of frontal sinus surgery in nasal polyp recurrence. Laryngoscope. 2013;123(1):36–41.
95. Ting JY, Wu A, Metson R. Frontal sinus drillout (modified Lothrop procedure): long-term results in 204 patients. Laryngoscope. 2014;124(5):1066–70.
96. Naidoo Y, Bassiouni A, Keen M, Wormald PJ. Long-term outcomes for the endoscopic modified Lothrop/Draf III procedure: a 10-year review. Laryngoscope. 2014;124(1):43–9.
97. Tran KN, Beule AG, Singal D, Wormald PJ. Frontal ostium restenosis after the endoscopic modified Lothrop procedure. Laryngoscope. 2007;117(8):1457–62.
98. Wong EH, Do TQ, Harvey RJ, Orgain CA, Sacks R, Kalish L. Patient-reported olfaction improves following outside-in Draf III frontal sinus surgery for chronic rhinosinusitis. Laryngoscope. 2019;129(1):25–30.

99. Patel VS, Choby G, Shih LC, Patel ZM, Nayak JV, Hwang PH. Equivalence in outcomes between Draf 2B vs Draf 3 frontal sinusotomy for refractory chronic frontal rhinosinusitis. Int Forum Allergy Rhinol. 2018;8(1):25–31.
100. McMains KC, Kountakis SE. Medical and surgical considerations in patients with Samter's triad. Am J Rhinol. 2006;20(6):573–6.
101. Cho KS, Soudry E, Psaltis AJ, Nadeau KC, McGhee SA, Nayak JV, et al. Long-term sinonasal outcomes of aspirin desensitization in aspirin exacerbated respiratory disease. Otolaryngol Head Neck Surg. 2014;151(4):575–81.
102. Glicksman JT, Parasher AK, Doghramji L, Brauer D, Waldram J, Walters K, et al. Alcohol-induced respiratory symptoms improve after aspirin desensitization in patients with aspirin-exacerbated respiratory disease. Int Forum Allergy Rhinol. 2018;8(10):1093–7.

Chapter 8
Cystic Fibrosis and Chronic Rhinosinusitis: Diagnosis and Medical Management

Kasper Aanaes

> **Key Concepts**
> - Cystic fibrosis (CF) is an autosomal recessive disease caused by mutations in the CF transmembrane conductance regulator (CFTR) protein.
> - CF patients may have advanced sinus disease even in the absence of symptoms.
> - Bacteria from the upper airway result in colonization, infection, and morbidity of the lower airway.

Description of Disorder

Cystic fibrosis (CF) is an autosomal recessive disease caused by mutations in the cystic fibrosis transmembrane conductance regulator (CFTR) protein located on chromosome 7 [1]. More than 1500 mutations in the gene have been found causing different clinical manifestations of the disease; the most frequently observed mutation is the ΔF508. The mutations are divided into six classes ranging from the severe total lack of functional CFTR synthesis to decreased stability of the CFTR channels.

K. Aanaes (✉)
Department of Otorhinolaryngology Head and Neck Surgery and Audiology,
Copenhagen University Hospital Rigshospitalet, Copenhagen, Denmark

© Springer Nature Switzerland AG 2020
D. A. Gudis, R. J. Schlosser (eds.), *The Unified Airway*,
https://doi.org/10.1007/978-3-030-50330-7_8

Epidemiology

CF is the most frequent lethal autosomal recessive disorder in the Caucasian population, but it affects all races. Ireland and the Faroe Islands have the highest prevalence of CF in the world with prevalence of, respectively, 68 per 100,000 (1:1461) in Ireland [2] and 56 per 100,000 (1:1775) in the Faroe Islands [3]. Within the white population in the United States, the disease occurs in 1 in approximately 3000 newborns. Cystic fibrosis is less common in other ethnic groups, affecting about 1 in 17,000 African Americans and 1 in 31,000 Asian Americans. One in 29 people of Caucasian ancestry is an unaffected carrier of the CF gene mutation [4].

Etiology and Pathogenesis

The CFTR gene encodes the cAMP-dependent chloride channel, and as a consequence of the defect, abnormal transport of chloride and sodium across the cell epithelium is seen. Thus, all secretions except sweat contain a lower concentration of salt, which more than doubles the viscosity compared with non-CF individuals [5]. The mucus is thus dehydrated and sticky, which reduces mucociliary clearance and promotes infections. This mucociliary dysfunction leads to increased susceptibility to bacterial infections in the lower airways with the CF-pathogenic gram-negative bacteria, particularly *Pseudomonas aeruginosa*, *Achromobacter xylosoxidans*, and *Burkholderia cepacia*; the biofilm-producing mucoid *P. aeruginosa* causes the most morbidity and mortality in CF patients. Methicillin-resistant strains of *Staphylococcus aureus* are also frequently encountered, and their presence is associated with worsening progression of lung disease.

The main clinical characteristics of CF are increased salt loss in sweat, malabsorption, diabetes, male infertility, chronic rhinosinusitis, and increased fungal and viral airway infections. The most severe clinical finding is the increased susceptibility to bacterial infections of the lower airways, resulting in a destructive inflammatory process. Thus, a hallmark of treating patients with CF is to prevent or delay chronic lung infections with CF-pathogenic gram-negative bacteria. Preventing chronic lung infections is, however, difficult to achieve, and the vast majority of patients with CF have been chronically infected or are even status post lung transplant by adulthood [6].

In the intermittently colonized lung stage preceding chronic infection, these bacteria are found in less than 50% of lower airway cultures. These bacteria can usually be eradicated from the lungs with inhaled and intravenous antibiotics. However, subsequent lung colonization following eradication often occurs with bacteria of identical genotype [7, 8], suggesting that the paranasal sinuses may serve as a reservoir for these bacterial colonies.

Nasal and sinus mucosal disease is by definition present in patients with CF [9] because of defective CFTR channels in the sinonasal and pulmonary mucosa. Only 7% of CF patients are free from inflammatory changes in their sinonasal histology

Fig. 8.1 Sticky secretions that are cleansed with difficulty during general anesthesia

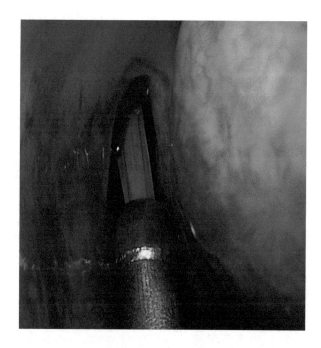

Fig. 8.2 A view of the nasal cavity from Fig. 8.3 showing nasal polyps

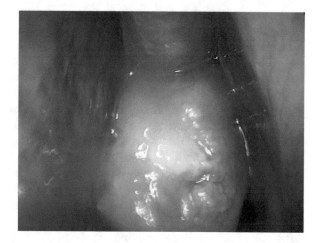

[10]. The inflamed tissue and sticky viscous mucus (Fig. 8.1) result in chronic rhinosinusitis (CRS) with or without nasal polyps. Nasal polyps in CF tend to be more neutrophilic and less eosinophilic compared to the non-CF population [11] but are macroscopically identical (Fig. 8.2).

In contrast to non-CF patients, virulent bacteria are more frequently present, and *P. aeruginosa* is the most common to colonize the sinuses and lungs in older CF patients. Other frequently found bacteria are *S. aureus*, *Haemophilus influenzae*, and coagulase-negative staphylococci. Anaerobes and other pathogenic gram-negative bacteria found in the lower airways such as *A. xylosoxidans* and *B. cepacia* complex are also found in the CF sinuses [12]. Presence of sinus bacteria is reported in 44–95% of CF patients [13–15]. Two articles have described fungal sinusitis among North American CF patients but disagree on the prevalence (0–33%) [15, 16].

Clinical Presentation

Patient Demographic and Medical Context

The male:female ratio is close to 1. The majority of patients with CF are diagnosed within their first year of life. CF patients seldom have a need for ENT consultation the first 5 years of life, likely because chronic otitis media is rare in this population and the paranasal sinuses are not yet developed. As the CF life expectancy has significantly increased over the last few decades, the majority of CF patients now are adolescents or adults.

Signs and Symptoms

There is no specific definition of chronic rhinosinusitis (CRS) in CF patients, so the general definition stated in the European Position Paper on Rhinosinusitis (EPOS) [9] is used. The inflamed tissue and viscous mucus result in a mechanical obstruction of the sinus ostia [17]. CRS can be present with or without nasal polyposis; bilateral nasal polyposis in children is often a clinical indication of CF [18]. Nasal polyposis becomes more common with age and has been reported in varying prevalence with up to 50% of all CF patients. Symptoms of CRS include thick nasal discharge, postnasal discharge, nasal blockage, facial pressure, and decreased sense of smell [19]. Approximately two-thirds of all CF patients have impaired olfactory function [20]. There is a strong association between nutritional status and pulmonary function in CF, and a decreased sense of smell is known to influence nutritional status in non-CF patients.

CF patients are likely to underreport their symptoms of CRS, suggesting a falsely low portion of CF patients with CRS. While only 10–15% of CF patients complain of CRS without specific questioning, 81–86% of CF patients fulfill the EPOS criteria [13, 21, 22]. It is unknown whether the CF patients who do not complain about CRS were always asymptomatic, if they have adapted to their symptoms, or if their CRS symptoms are overshadowed by more troublesome symptoms from, for example, their pulmonary disease [23]. Individuals who are carriers of one defective CFTR gene may be more predisposed to developing CRS.

Nonspecific symptoms such as cough, lack of a good night's sleep, and fatigue can all originate from the upper airways as well as from the lower airways. Pulmonologists who care for CF patients should regularly ask them about symptoms of lower airway infections, including severe cough, fever, difficulty breathing, rapid breathing, and wheezing. Furthermore, CF patients' lung function should be closely monitored with percent predicted lung function, and regular cultures should be obtained by expectorated sputum, endolaryngeal suction, induced sputum, or bronchoalveolar lavage (four to twelve times per year). Specific anti-*Pseudomonas* IgG or IgA antibodies measured by ELISA [24] and precipitating antibodies measured by crossed immunoelectrophoresis [25] are all methods which can be used when evaluating the CF patient's infection status.

Diagnostics

Characteristic Physical Exam and Nasal Endoscopy Findings

Cystic fibrosis is often diagnosed at birth. In several countries, neonatal screening is performed within the first couple of days of life. If the screening test is positive, a genetic test and sweat chloride test are performed. A genetic test is often offered to the partner of a patient with cystic fibrosis if children are considered. Early detection and thereby early treatment can prevent malnutrition and delay lung infections.

The Cystic Fibrosis Questionnaire-Revised (CFQ-R) is a commonly used questionnaire to estimate the disease-specific health-related quality of life [26], but it does not evaluate sinonasal symptoms. When specifically asked, CF patients are often quite good at describing the characteristic pressure caused by sinusitis, which changes with head positions and has specific anatomic locations (the forehead, cheek area, behind the eyes, or midface). The Sinonasal Outcome Test-22 (SNOT-22) is used worldwide when evaluating CRS [27] but also includes health-related questions that can be influenced by other CF-related conditions.

All CF patients with sinonasal symptoms should be evaluated by an otolaryngologist experienced in sinonasal disease management. Routine exam should include nasal endoscopy, where the doctor may identify mucosal edema or nasal polyps, which may appear similar to polyps in non-CF patients [3]. Thick secretions or pus from the middle meatus draining posteriorly to the rhinopharynx is a common finding. A swab or nasal irrigation for culture should be done, but one should be aware that, especially in patients who have not had sinus surgery, the culture can be false negative for pathogenic bacteria. As in the lungs, the sinuses can be noninfected or chronically infected where the bacteria are nearly impossible to eradicate despite surgery and antibiotics; in between these subtypes is a broad stage of intermittent sinonasal colonization ranging from bacteria (e.g., *P. aeruginosa*) detected only by molecular methods, to the presence of sparse intramucosal pus and bacteria in some sinuses, to visible thick pus in nearly all sinuses.

Fig. 8.3 CT scan showing total opacified nasal cavity and sinuses. Naturally, this patient had a lot of upper airway symptoms

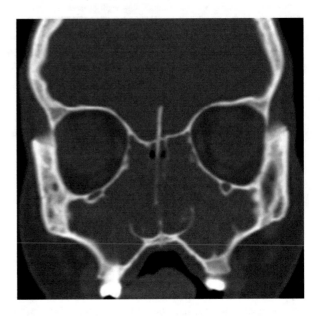

Fig. 8.4 CT scan showing a patient previously having sinus surgery; inspite of accessible maxillary sinuses they are opacifed due to mucosal edema

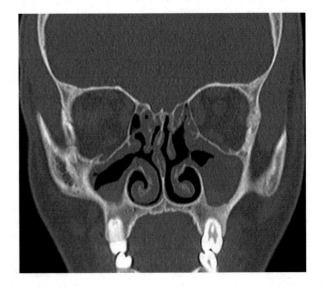

Typical CT Radiographic Features

Anatomically, CF patients often have hypoplastic sinuses, independent of previous surgery. A study on adult CF patients demonstrated that 66% of the frontal sinuses were either aplastic or hypoplastic [28]. Mucoceles often leading to pyoceles and bone sclerosis are common, as well as typical inflammatory patterns, e.g., sinonasal polyposis, mucosal swelling and bulging, or even absence of the lateral nasal wall

[28] (Figs. 8.3 and 8.4). The vast majority of CF patients have radiologic evidence of sinus disease and characteristic CT findings from early childhood [29]; thus, the Lund-Mackay scoring system may not be optimal. Alternative CT sinus scoring systems addressing CF [30–32] may be more useful since mucosal swelling is very common and can be specified. To minimize radiation exposure, CT scans should not be performed routinely. Indications for CT include consideration of surgery, symptom recurrence postoperatively, or concern for a complication of sinusitis.

Medical Management and Outcomes

Systemic Medical Therapy

As no cure exists for CF, the management of CF CRS is currently based on patients' symptoms and treatment of the underlying gene defect. In non-CF patients with refractory CRS, systemic antibiotics and corticosteroids have great efficacy in reducing the amount of secretions and polyp burden. Unfortunately, these treatments may not be as effective in CF patients. Systemic steroids are thought to be less effective in CF patients because their sinonasal mucosal disease is a TH1 neutrophilic inflammation. There are no studies investigating the impact of systemic steroids on sinonasal symptoms in CF patients. Furthermore, systemic antibiotics without surgical drainage are not thought to be efficacious.

In recent years, new CFTR potentiator drugs have been developed. Ivacaftor increases the opening probability of the CFTR channels at the cell surface, thus increasing the flow of ions through the channel. Ivacaftor has been shown to improve CRS symptoms in some CF patients. More CFTR modulator drugs and studies demonstrating their efficacy are expected in the future.

Topical Medical Therapy

The use of topical nasal corticosteroids is debated and the level of evidence is low. Nevertheless, since side effects of nasal steroids are rare, they are often used, and some patients do report improved sinonasal symptoms after use. As in non-CF CRS patients, to relieve sinonasal symptoms, nasal irrigations should always be tried prior to surgical intervention [33]. There is high-level evidence that nasal irrigations with saline relieve symptoms in CF patients, and the procedure is well tolerated in all ages.

Nasal irrigation can be combined with dornase alfa to loosen sinonasal secretions. Dornase alfa inhaled as vibrating aerosol has been shown to be even more effective than nasal saline irrigation alone [34]. The use of topical antibiotics also correlates with improvement in symptom and endoscopic scoring [35, 36]. Nevertheless, when CF patients have severe sinonasal symptoms and radiographic evidence of advanced disease, medical management is often inadequate to improve their CRS.

Surgical Management

Criteria for Surgery

There is a high concordance between bacteria cultured from the paranasal sinuses and from the lungs [7, 37–39]. There is lower bioavailability of intravenous antibiotic treatment in the sinuses compared to the lungs [40, 41]. It has been shown that *P. aeruginosa* over time develops phenotypic traits and mutations (e.g., biofilm formation) in the sinuses before they are identified in the lungs, making them more resistant to eradication. Infections often originate in the paranasal sinuses and can then be responsible for initial and recurrent lung colonization [7, 38, 39]. Therefore, when the sinuses are colonized, sinus surgery should be considered. Urgent sinus treatment might be necessary to avoid chronic lung infections, improve lung function, and reduce pulmonary morbidity. Sinus surgery should also be considered in CF patients with early lung colonization of *P. aeruginosa* or other gram-negative bacteria, in hopes of eradicating these bacteria from the sinuses. However, there is a lack of diagnostic tools to detect early colonization in the lungs and in the sinuses. Therefore, in our practice, there are four primary indications for sinus surgery:

- In intermittently lung-colonized CF patients with the following:
  - Positive nasal culture showing gram-negative bacteria, e.g., *P. aeruginosa*
  - Increasing frequency of positive lower airway cultures or repeatedly declining lung function (>10%), despite intensive antibiotic chemotherapy
  - Increasing antibodies against *P. aeruginosa*, *A. xylosoxidans*, or *B. cepacia* complex

- In chronically lung-infected CF patients with good lung function, indicating that positive cultures and/or increasing antibodies are caused by upper airway bacteria
- In patients who have recently undergone lung transplantation
- In patients with severe symptoms of CRS, including patients who have already undergone surgery and require revision

Surgical Approach

The surgeon should be familiar with the anatomic features of CF sinuses. When doing surgery in an attempt to eradicate bacteria, it should be noted that bacteria can be identified and cultured in all sinuses, including those that appear clear on CT. Therefore, surgery should be comprehensive and address all sinuses. Some surgeons scrape the mucosa intraoperatively and perform repeated perioperative irrigations to remove all entrapped purulent secretions. Several studies have demonstrated improved outcomes with extended surgery, including total ethmoidectomy, medial maxillectomy [42], and Draf 2B procedures. Sinus osteoneogenesis and bony sclerosis may make the surgery more challenging.

Impact of Rhinologic Interventions

Endoscopic sinus surgery in CF children and adults is a safe procedure despite anatomic variations in this population [43]. Several unambiguous reports have shown
that sinus surgery reduces sinonasal symptoms in CF patients. One study comprising 106 CF patients showed that despite a revision rate of 28% within 3 years,
patients still had a significant reduction in symptoms and often had a strong desire
for surgery [44].

Several studies have evaluated the effect of sinus surgery on pulmonary outcomes with divergent conclusions. However, only two prospective studies have
been performed that addressed all the sinuses with the goal of eradicating bacteria:
one focused on a large cohort of lung-transplanted CF patients and found reduced
bronchiolitis obliterans syndrome after sinus surgery [45]; the other focused on a
large heterogeneous CF population and found a reduced number of CF patients
becoming chronically lung-infected after sinus surgery [44]. When evaluating these
studies, it is important to consider the preoperative lung infection status, the extent
of sinus surgery, and the postoperative adjuvant medical treatment and to keep in
mind that the natural course of CF is declining lung function.

With regard to postsurgical treatment, most studies use topical and/or systemic
antibiotic therapy, similar to the well-established pulmonary treatment protocols
of inhaled antibiotics. However, recurrent sinus infections are often seen. In the
future, instillation of resorbable antibiotics, CFTR-modulating drugs, and other
novel therapies may show a beneficial effect on eradicating the pathogenic bacteria
after surgery [46–48].

Case Presentation

An 11-year-old boy homozygous with delta F508 CF mutations was seen in our
ENT department. In the previous 8 months, four out of seven sputum cultures taken
by suction from the lower airways cultured positive for non-mucoid *Pseudomonas
aeruginosa*. His blood samples showed increased precipitating *Pseudomonas
aeruginosa* antibodies. His lung function test had decreased from 103 to 96 percent of predicted value within the same period of time. At this rate, he would
satisfy our definition of chronically lung-infected if this pattern continued for four
more months.

Endoscopic examination did not show any visible polyps or pus. A culture from
the middle meatus showed only coagulase-negative staphylococci. A CT scan was
taken (Fig. 8.5) showing total opacification of the left frontal sinus with surrounding
neo-osteogenesis, some general mucosal edema, and hypoplasia of the right frontal
sinus and both sphenoid sinuses.

Endoscopic sinus surgery was performed, finding polyps and thick sticky secretions within the maxillary sinuses and pus in the left frontal sinus later culturing

Fig. 8.5 CT scan showing opacification of the left frontal sinus and a right hypoplastic right frontal sinus

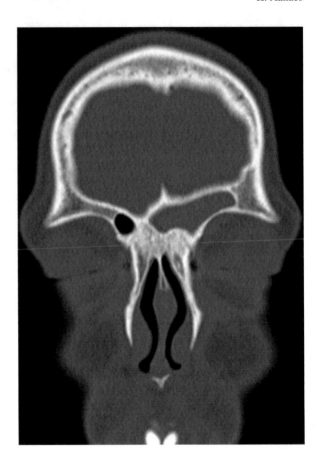

positive for *P. aeruginosa*. All sinuses were addressed (including a Draf 1 frontal sinusotomy due to hypoplasia and no medial maxillectomy), and the sinuses were then irrigated with colistin. The boy had 14 days of IV antibiotics and did 3 months of nasal irrigations with saline combined with colistin and topical nasal steroids.

With monthly postoperative cultures from the lower airways, *P. aeruginosa* was not cultured again until 480 days postoperatively. The patient underwent revision sinus surgery 2.5 years later, revealing *P. aeruginosa* in several sinuses.

This patient demonstrates the capacity of sinus surgery and adjuvant medical therapy to reduce positive *P. aeruginosa* pulmonary cultures. His surgery was remarkable in that the purulence in his frontal sinus was under so much pressure that pus squirted out the nose all the way down to his belly (Fig. 8.6). His SNOT-22 score (range 0–110) was not high but decreased from 18 preoperatively to 9 three months postoperatively.

Fig. 8.6 Pus in the middle meatus during surgery

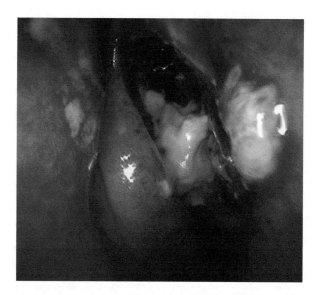

Conclusion

Cystic fibrosis is a troublesome and complex disease that clearly demonstrates the unified airway concept. In contrast to patients with asthma, CF patients may have advanced sinonasal disease even in the absence of symptoms. However, it is evident that secretions and bacteria from the upper airways are transported to the lower airways resulting in pulmonary colonization, symptoms, and morbidity. Pulmonologists should ask patients with cystic fibrosis about upper airway symptoms and consider the sinuses as a bacterial reservoir and source of pulmonary infections. Otolaryngologists should collaborate closely with pulmonologists in the comprehensive management of CF patients.

References

1. Kerem B, Rommens JM, Buchanan JA, Markiewicz D, Cox TK, Chakravarti A, et al. Identification of the cystic fibrosis gene: genetic analysis. Science. 1989;245(4922):1073–80.
2. Cashman SM, Patino A, Delgado MG, Byrne L, Denham B, De Arce M. The Irish cystic fibrosis database. J Med Genet. 1995;32:972–5.
3. Schwartz M, Sørensen N, Brandt NJ, Høgdall E, Holm T. High incidence of cystic fibrosis on The Faroe Islands: a molecular and genealogical study. Hum Genet. 1995;95:703–6.
4. https://www.thoracic.org/patients/patient-resources/breathing-in-america/resources/chapter-7-cystic-fibrosis.pdf
5. Doggett RG, Harrision GM, Wallis ES. Comparison of some properties of Pseudomonas aeruginosa isolated from infections in persons with and without cystic fibrosis. J Bacteriol. 1964;87:427–31.

6. Lyczak JB, Cannon CL, Pier GB. Lung infections associated with cystic fibrosis. Clin Microbiol Rev. 2002;15:194–222.
7. Mainz JG, Naehrlich L, Schien M, et al. Concordant genotype of upper and lower airways P aeruginosa and S aureus isolates in cystic fibrosis. Thorax. 2009;64:535–40.
8. Hansen SK, Rau MH, Johansen HK, Ciofu O, Jelsbak L, Yang L, et al. Evolution and diversification of Pseudomonas aeruginosa in the paranasal sinuses of cystic fibrosis children have implications for chronic lung infection. ISME J. 2012;6(1):31–45.
9. Fokkens WJ, Lund VJ, Mullol J, Bachert C, Alobid I, Baroody F, et al. EPOS 2012: European position paper on rhinosinusitis and nasal polyps 2012. A summary for otorhinolaryngologists. Rhinology. 2012;50(1):1–12.
10. Babinski D, Trawinska-Bartnicka M. Rhinosinusitis in cystic fibrosis: not a simple story. Int J Pediatr Otorhinolaryngol. 2008;72:619–24.
11. Steinke JW, Payne SC, Chen PG, Negri J, Stelow EB, Borish L. Etiology of nasal polyps in cystic fibrosis: not a unimodal disease. Ann Otol Rhinol Laryngol. 2012;121:579–86.
12. Møller ME, Alanin MC, Grønhøj C, Aanæs K, Høiby N, von Buchwald C. Sinus bacteriology in patients with cystic fibrosis or primary ciliary dyskinesia: a systematic review. Am J Rhinol Allergy. 2107;31(5):293–8.
13. Bonestroo HJ, de Winter-de Groot KM, van der Ent CK, Arets HG. Upper and lower airway cultures in children with cystic fibrosis: do not neglect the upper airways. J Cyst Fibros. 2010;9(2):130–4.
14. Shapiro ED, Milmoe GJ, Wald ER, Rodnan JB, Bowen AD. Bacteriology of the maxillary sinuses in patients with cystic fibrosis. J Infect Dis. 1982;146(5):589–93.
15. Roby BB, McNamara J, Finkelstein M, Sidman J. Sinus surgery in cystic fibrosis patients: comparison of sinus and lower airway cultures. Int J Pediatr Otorhinolaryngol. 2008;72(9):1365–9.
16. Wise SK, Kingdom TT, McKean L, DelGaudio JM, Venkatraman G. Presence of fungus in sinus cultures of cystic fibrosis patients. Am J Rhinol. 2005;19(1):47–51.
17. Loebinger MR, Bilton D, Wilson R. Upper airway 2: bronchiectasis, cystic fibrosis and sinusitis. Thorax. 2009;64(12):1096–101.
18. Marshak T, Rivlin Y, Bentur L, Ronen O, Uri N. Prevalence of rhinosinusitis among atypical cystic fibrosis patients. Eur Arch Otorhinolaryngol. 2011;268:519–24.
19. Bock JM, Schien M, Fischer C, et al. Importance to question sinonasal symptoms and to perform rhinoscopy and rhinomanometry in cystic fibrosis patients. Pediatr Pulmonol. 2017;52:167–74.
20. Lindig J, Steger C, Beiersdorf N, Michl R, Beck JF, Hummel T, et al. Smell in cystic fibrosis. Eur Arch Otorhinolaryngol. 2013;270(3):915–21.
21. Berkhout MC, van Rooden CJ, Rijntjes E, Fokkens WJ, el Bouazzaoui LH, Heijerman HG. Sinonasal manifestations of cystic fibrosis: a correlation between genotype and phenotype? J Cyst Fibros. 2014;13:442–8.
22. King VV. Upper respiratory disease, sinusitis, and polyposis. Clin Rev Allergy. 1991;9(1–2):143–57.
23. Robertson JM, Friedman EM, Rubin BK. Nasal and sinus disease in cystic fibrosis. Paediatr Respir Rev. 2008;9(3):213–9.
24. Pressler T, Frederiksen B, Skov M, Garred P, Koch C, Hoiby N. Early rise of anti-pseudomonas antibodies and a mucoid phenotype of pseudomonas aeruginosa are risk factors for development of chronic lung infection--a case control study. J Cyst Fibros. 2006;5(1):9–15.
25. Johansen HK, Norregaard L, Gotzsche PC, Pressler T, Koch C, Hoiby N. Antibody response to Pseudomonas aeruginosa in cystic fibrosis patients: a marker of therapeutic success?--a 30-year cohort study of survival in Danish CF patients after onset of chronic P. aeruginosa lung infection. Pediatr Pulmonol. 2004;37(5):427–32.
26. Quittner AL, Buu A, Messer MA, Modi AC, Watrous M. Development and validation of the cystic fibrosis questionnaire in the United States: a health-related quality-of-life measure for cystic fibrosis. Chest. 2005;128(4):2347–54.
27. Hopkins C, Gillett S, Slack R, Lund VJ, Browne JP. Psychometric validity of the 22-item sinonasal outcome test. Clin Otolaryngol. 2009;34(5):447–54.

28. Orlandi RR, Wiggins RH. Radiological sinonasal findings in adults with cystic fibrosis. Am J Rhinol Allergy. 2009;23:307–11.
29. Berkhout MC, Klerx-Melis F, Fokkens WJ, Nuijsink M, van Aalderen WM, Heijerman HG. CT-abnormalities, bacteriology and symptoms of sinonasal disease in children with cystic fibrosis. J Cyst Fibros. 2016;15:816–24.
30. Eggesbo HB, Sovik S, Dolvik S, Eiklid K, Kolmannskog F. Proposal of a CT scoring system of the paranasal sinuses in diagnosing cystic fibrosis. Eur Radiol. 2003;13:1451–60.
31. Sheikh SI, Handly B, Ryan-Wenger NA, et al. Novel computed tomography scoring system for sinus disease in adults with cystic fibrosis. Ann Otol Rhinol Laryngol. 2016;125:838–43.
32. Rasmussen J, Aanaes K, Norling R, Nielsen KG, Johansen HK, von Buchwald C. CT of the paranasal sinuses is not a valid indicator for sinus surgery in CF patients. J Cyst Fibros. 2012;11:93–9.
33. Ayoub N, Thamboo A, Habib A-R, Nayak JV, Hwang PH. Determinants and outcomes of upfront surgery versus medical therapy for chronic rhinosinusitis in cystic fibrosis. Int Forum Allergy Rhinol. 2017;7:450–8.
34. Cimmino M, Nardone M, Cavaliere M, et al. Dornase alfa as postoperative therapy in cystic fibrosis sinonasal disease. Arch Otolaryngol Head Neck Surg. 2005;131:1097–101.
35. Lee VS, Davis GE. Culture-directed topical antibiotic treatment for chronic rhinosinusitis. Am J Rhinol Allergy. 2016;30:414–7.
36. Berkhout MC, van Velzen AJ, Touw DJ, de Kok BM, Fokkens WJ, Heijerman HGM. Systemic absorption of nasally administered tobramycin and colistin in patients with cystic fibrosis. J Antimicrob Chemother. 2014;69:3112–5.
37. Aanaes K, Johansen HK, Skov M, et al. Clinical effects of sinus surgery and adjuvant therapy in cystic fibrosis patients – can chronic lung infections be postponed? Rhinology. 2013;51:222–30.
38. Markussen T, Marvig RL, Gómez-Lozano M, et al. Environmental heterogeneity drives within-host diversification and evolution of pseudomonas aeruginosa. MBio. 2014;5:e01592–14.
39. Pletcher SD, Goldberg AN, Cope EK. Loss of microbial niche specificity between the upper and lower airways in patients with cystic fibrosis. Laryngoscope. 2019;129:544–50.
40. Doht F, Hentschel J, Fischer N, et al. Reduced effect of intravenous antibiotic treatment on sinonasal markers in pulmonary inflammation. Rhinology. 2015;53:249–59.
41. Johansen HK, Aanaes K, Pressler T, et al. Colonisation and infection of the paranasal sinuses in cystic fibrosis patients is accompanied by a reduced PMN response. J Cyst Fibros. 2012;11:525–31.
42. Virgin FW, Rowe SM, Wade MB, et al. Extensive surgical and comprehensive postoperative medical management for cystic fibrosis chronic rhinosinusitis. Am J Rhinol Allergy. 2012;26:70–5.
43. Tumin D, Hayes D, Kirkby SE, Tobias JD, McKee C. Safety of endoscopic sinus surgery in children with cystic fibrosis. Int J Pediatr Otorhinolaryngol. 2017;98:25–8.
44. Alanin MC, Aanaes K, Hoiby N, et al. Sinus surgery postpones chronic gram-negative lung infection: cohort study of 106 patients with cystic fibrosis. Rhinology. 2016;54:206–13.
45. Vital D, Hofer M, Benden C, Holzmann D, Boehler A. Impact of sinus surgery on pseudomonal airway colonization, bronchiolitis obliterans syndrome and survival in cystic fibrosis lung transplant recipients. Respiration. 2013;86:25–31.
46. Cho DY, Lim DJ, Mackey C, et al. In-vitro evaluation of a ciprofloxacin- and ivacaftor-coated sinus stent against Pseudomonas aeruginosa biofilms. Int Forum Allergy Rhinol. 2019;9:486–92.
47. Fong SA, Drilling A, Morales S, et al. Activity of bacteriophages in removing biofilms of pseudomonas aeruginosa isolates from chronic rhinosinusitis patients. Front Cell Infect Microbiol. 2017;7:418.
48. Hashemi MM, Holden BS, Taylor MF, et al. Antibacterial and antifungal activities of poloxamer micelles containing ceragenin CSA-131 on ciliated tissues. Molecules (Basel, Switzerland). 2018;23:596.

Chapter 9
Cystic Fibrosis and Chronic Rhinosinusitis: Surgical Management and Outcomes

Daniel Spielman, Chetan Safi, Jonathan Overdevest, and David A. Gudis

> **Key Concepts**
> - Endoscopic sinus surgery for cystic fibrosis (CF) CRS can significantly improve sinonasal symptoms.
> - Extended surgical approaches can facilitate mucociliary clearance and topical medical therapy access.
> - Recent clinical trials have demonstrated that combined surgical and medical management for CF CRS improves CF pulmonary outcome measures.

Cystic fibrosis is caused by a mutation in the cystic fibrosis transmembrane conductance (CFTR) gene that leads to impaired chloride ion transport across cell membranes. Reduced chloride ion transport leads to poor osmosis of water and a resultant increase in thick, inspissated secretions, poor mucociliary clearance, and bacterial colonization [1]. This chronic inflammation of the respiratory epithelium leads to recurrent pulmonary exacerbations as well as chronic rhinosinusitis [2]. Furthermore, investigators have found that the paranasal sinuses in CF patients can serve as a reservoir for pathogenic bacteria that can lead to pulmonary exacerbations, adding more evidence to support the unified airway model [3–5]. Thus, it is key to develop an interdisciplinary treatment strategy to treat CF patients with a combination of medical and surgical therapy.

D. Spielman · C. Safi · J. Overdevest · D. A. Gudis (✉)
Department of Otolaryngology – Head & Neck Surgery, Columbia University Irving Medical Center, New York-Presbyterian Hospital, New York, NY, USA
e-mail: dag62@cumc.columbia.edu

© Springer Nature Switzerland AG 2020
D. A. Gudis, R. J. Schlosser (eds.), *The Unified Airway*,
https://doi.org/10.1007/978-3-030-50330-7_9

Clinical Presentation

The challenge in CF CRS is identifying those patients who have clinically relevant sinusitis requiring treatment. The International Consensus on Allergy and Rhinology states that CRS is defined by persistent sinus inflammation for over 12 weeks with the presence of subjective symptoms and objective findings [6]. However, in CF CRS, while 60–80% of patients will have radiographic evidence of mucosal inflammation, fewer than 20% will report symptoms without direct questioning [7]. However, most clinicians still use a combination of nasal endoscopy, computed tomography (CT), and quality of life (QOL) metrics to assess for sinonasal pathology in patients who endorse the classical symptoms of CRS such as nasal obstruction, facial pain, decreased sense of smell, and rhinorrhea [2, 6].

On nasal endoscopy, patients with CF CRS will often have evidence of thick nasal secretions and/or purulence as well as mucosal edema and nasal polyposis. To provide uniform data, these nasal endoscopy findings can be translated to a Lund-Kennedy nasal endoscopy (LKNE) score. Casserly et al. found that CF patients with and without subjective symptoms of CRS had similar LKNE scores, which were overall worse than the general population without CRS, indicating a clinically detectable increased level of sinonasal inflammation on nasal endoscopy in CF patients [8].

On computed tomography, findings of paranasal sinus hypoplasia/aplasia, medial bulging of the lateral nasal wall, demineralization of the uncinate process, sphenoethmoidal recess inflammation, sinus opacification, osteitis and neoosteo-genesis, and sclerosis of paranasal sinus bone are characteristic of CF CRS [9, 10]. Moreover, differing CF genotypes have been correlated with varying degrees of paranasal sinus development. One group found that patients with a homozygous delta F508 mutation are statistically more likely to have underdeveloped maxillary, frontal, and sphenoid sinuses as compared to those with other mutations [11]. However, CT imaging findings do not always correlate with patients' symptoms. For example, Kang et al. found that while 84.7% of a CF cohort had radiologic evidence of CRS, there was no statistical difference in Lund-MacKay scores among patients stratified by the severity of their Sinonasal Outcome Test-22 (SNOT-22) scores [9]. Furthermore, Rasmussen et al. state that the decision for endoscopic sinus surgery (ESS) should not be based solely on CT findings, as their study found purulence and pathogenic bacteria in patients without sinus opacification on CT and, conversely, sterile cultures in patients with sinus opacification on imaging [12].

The effect of CF CRS on a patient's quality of life can also help determine which patients have clinically relevant disease requiring treatment. Habib et al. found that a Sinonasal Outcome Test-22 (SNOT-22) score greater than 21 was indicative of CF CRS in CF patients. Moreover, the study found that SNOT-22, as a single variable predictor, did not differ from a multivariable regression model, including several sociodemographic and clinical variables, in determining the presence or absence of CRS [13]. Another study found that the respiratory component of the Cystic Fibrosis Questionnaire-Revised for adults and adolescents above age 14 (CFQ-R 14+) was statistically lower in patients with CRS compared to patients without CRS, indicating worsened perceived respiratory health in those with CRS [14]. Thus, these quality of life metrics, in combination with nasal endoscopy and CT, can be used to target patients who would benefit the most from aggressive medical and surgical therapy for CF CRS.

Medical Management and Outcomes

Many topical and systemic therapies to medically treat CF CRS have been identified in the literature. Dornase alfa cleaves extracellular DNA and is a mucolytic agent that improves lung function and reduces pulmonary exacerbations [15]. Cimmino et al. treated CF patients with 1 year of nasal nebulized dornase alfa therapy or placebo therapy after undergoing endoscopic sinus surgery. At 48 weeks after surgery, patients treated with dornase alfa had a statistically significant improvement in their sinonasal symptoms, LKNE score, Lund-Mackay score, and forced expiratory volume in 1 second (FEV1) [16]. Additionally, another study found that CF patients treated with intranasal dornase alfa had a statistically significant improvement in SNOT-22 scores as well as forced expiratory flow 25–75% when compared to patients using isotonic saline [17].

When considering saline irrigations, Mainz et al. performed a randomized clinical trial in which CF patients used both 28 days of isotonic saline irrigations and 28 days of hypertonic (6.0%) saline irrigations with a washout period in between. Both therapies led to similarly small improvements in SNOT-22 [18]. One possible explanation for this could be lack of adequate sinus penetration. Aanaes et al. found that even after ESS, no saline irrigation reached the frontal or sphenoid sinus while less than 50% of maxillary sinuses showed an increase in postoperative fluid volume with irrigations [19].

Topical corticosteroids are another option for the treatment of CF CRS. Hadfield et al. found that CF patients with nasal polyposis treated with twice daily beclomethasone for 6 weeks had reduction in nasal polyposis but no change in symptom score when compared to placebo [20]. Donaldson et al. found that 62.5% of CF patients with nasal polyposis had an improvement in their nasal polyposis and 78.6% of patients without nasal polyposis had improvement in nasal obstructive symptoms with twice daily nasal inhalation of beclomethasone totaling 100 mg [21].

Topical antibiotics have also been used by many physicians to treat sinus disease in CF patients. Aerosolized tobramycin resulted in a decrease of paranasal sinus P. aeruginosa growth as well as a statistically significant improvement in SNOT-20 scores when compared to placebo [22]. Moss et al. found that postoperative serial sinus lavage with antibiotics such as tobramycin after ESS resulted in a reoperative rate of 10% and 22% at 1 and 2 years postoperatively, respectively. Patients who underwent only ESS without topical tobramycin had a reoperation rate of 47% and 72% at 1 and 2 years, respectively [23].

Ivacaftor is a novel CFTR modulator that improves ion transport function in patients with a specific class of CFTR mutations called gating mutations. Its efficacy in pulmonary disease has been widely studied; however, the data on its use in CF CRS is limited. McCormick et al. demonstrated that ivacaftor therapy improved patients' rhinologic, sleep, and psychological domain scores on the SNOT-20 1 and 3 months after starting therapy [24]. Furthermore, Chang et al. described a patient with medically and surgically recalcitrant CF CRS that underwent 10 months of ivacaftor therapy, resulting in complete resolution of maxillary and frontal sinus disease, improved symptomatology, and improved FEV1 [25]. Though more robust data is currently lacking, it is possible that as more CFTR-modulating drugs are developed, longitudinal research may show an improvement in upper airway disease as well as lower airway disease.

Ibuprofen has also been described as a systemic therapy for CF-related sinonasal disease though the data is limited. One study showed that though high-dose ibuprofen led to resolution of nasal polyps in 12 patients, more than half of whom had a recurrence of nasal polyps after stopping therapy [26].

Surgical Management and Outcomes

Functional endoscopic sinus surgery (FESS) is indicated in patients with persistent CRS despite maximal medical therapy. While there are no definitive established indications for surgery in the management of CF CRS, Ayoub et al. demonstrate that patients who underwent surgery had higher rates of nasal polyposis as well as higher Lund-Mackay and SNOT-22 scores preoperatively but a lower FEV1 score [27].

As compared to patients without CF, patients with CF CRS experience similar improvements in quality of life score and postoperative endoscopy after undergoing endoscopic sinus surgery [28].

Many studies have documented the efficacy of surgery in managing CF CRS. The cumulative results of these studies are captured in two major systematic reviews by Liang et al. and Macdonald et al. assessing outcomes of more than 500 patients with CF CRS who underwent surgery in addition to maximal medical therapy. These studies reveal that sinus surgery is safe in patients with CF CRS and results in improvement in subjective patient-reported symptoms [29, 30]. The majority of studies also noted improvement in objective nasal endoscopy scores postoperatively. Importantly, delaying surgery does not appear to limit postoperative improvement [28].

Patients with CF CRS typically have pansinusitis due to the systemic etiology of their condition. As such, when surgery is indicated, all paranasal sinuses are addressed. Cultures should be obtained in the operating room to guide postoperative antibiotic therapy. Careful review of preoperative sinus CT scan is essential to prevent complications, as CF patients are more likely to have low sloping ethmoid roof, which may increase the risk of intraoperative skull base complication [31].

Patients with CF CRS are also more likely to require revision sinus surgery. Published rates are highly variable, with several studies reporting revision rates between 29% and 52% [32, 33]. No difference in revision rates was found based on genetic subtype of CF [32]. Preoperative grade of polyposis correlates with likelihood of undergoing revision surgery. In one study, patients with high-grade polyposis were significantly more likely to require revision surgery at a rate of 58% with a shorter time to relapse (23.8 months) [33]. Because of the high rates of revision surgery and significantly impaired mucociliary clearance, some advocate for more aggressive surgery at initial intervention. At a minimum, this includes complete FESS with removal of all ethmoid partitions. For patients with significant frontal sinus disease, modified Lothrop procedure may be indicated [34]. Virgin et al. advocate for modified endoscopic medial maxillectomy to promote gravity-dependent drainage [35]. The superior location of the maxillary ostium can result in significant mucous stasis even with an enlarged antrostomy.

Impact of CF CRS Management on Pulmonary Disease

Recognizing the strong connection between the upper and lower airways, many studies have investigated the effects of CRS management, particularly sinus surgery, on lower airway outcomes. Several studies have demonstrated that comprehensive CRS treatment including ESS and postoperative topical antibiotic sinus irrigations reduces sinonasal colonization of pathogenic bacteria and delays gram-negative pulmonary infections [36, 37].

However, multiple metrics have been evaluated to determine the effects of sinus surgery on lung function with variable outcomes. Several studies document decreased inpatient hospitalization days in the 6 months following sinus surgery [35, 38–40]. Two studies have found that sinus surgery decreases the need for future IV antibiotics [38, 41].

The relationship between CRS management and pulmonary function is not clear in the CF population. Kovell et al. report improvement in postoperative pulmonary function testing after sinus surgery [42]. However, this finding is controversial and has been refuted by multiple other studies [39, 40].

A study by Holzmann et al. examined the effect of sinus surgery with comprehensive medical management in CF patients' status-post lung transplant. Successful sinus management led to a lower incidence of tracheobronchitis and pneumonia. Over 80% of patients had "successful" or "partially successful" resolution of their sinusitis as defined by the rates of positive bacterial cultures. This correlated significantly with negative bronchoalveolar lavage [43]. This finding is especially important, affirming the close connection between the upper and lower airways. Vital et al. also investigated the effects of comprehensive CRS management in the post-transplant patient population, successfully eradicating pseudomonal colonization in one-third of patients with pretransplant colonization. This finding was associated with decreased rates of bronchiolitis obliterans and improved survival [44]. These studies affirm the importance of sinonasal evaluation in the CF lung transplant population, including in those without significant sinonasal symptoms.

Case Presentation

Abbie is a 26-year-old Caucasian female with cystic fibrosis (homozygous delta F508 mutation) diagnosed soon after birth. She is referred by her pulmonologist for evaluation of her sinuses. Past medical history is notable for several hospitalizations for pneumonia, ultimately leading to profound lung disease requiring bilateral lung transplantation 2 years prior. Since that time, her respiratory symptoms are significantly improved, but she reports near lifelong facial pressure, hyposmia, and postnasal drip. Her SNOT-22 score is 44. She has been prescribed many courses of antibiotics for sinus symptoms and uses a nasal steroid spray and nasal saline rinses. Her symptoms have progressively worsened over the last 2 years.

Her physical exam reveals a well-appearing woman breathing comfortably at rest on room air. Nasal endoscopy reveals midline intact septum. She has bilateral inferior turbinate hypertrophy. There is bilateral nasal polyposis in the middle meatus with thick mucopurulent secretions. Nasopharynx examination reveals tenacious mucopurulent postnasal discharge.

A CT sinus is obtained, demonstrating pan-sinus opacification with osteitic bone. The maxillary and frontal sinuses are hypoplastic. There is no bony dehiscence of the lamina papyracea, anterior skull base, or sphenoid sinus. A representative image is demonstrated in Fig. 9.1.

The patient is offered continued medical therapy versus a combination of medical and surgical therapy. She understands that surgery is merely one component of treatment, which will allow improved access of topical therapy to enter the sinuses.

Fig. 9.1 CT sinus is obtained but shows no bony dehiscence of the lamina papyracea, anterior skull base, or sphenoid sinus

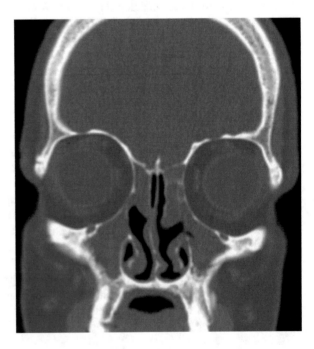

Fig. 9.2 The patient continues to use medicated irrigations and follows up at 3-month intervals for surveillance, with significant improvement in her nasal endoscopy

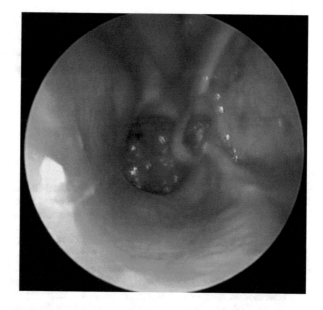

Abbie is interested in surgery due to her disease progression despite intranasal steroids, antibiotics, and saline rinses.

Surgery is planned in a multidisciplinary center. Abbie receives preoperative anesthesiology and pulmonary evaluations to optimize her care. FESS including bilateral modified endoscopic medial maxillectomies is performed to remove nasal polyposis, drain and culture the sinuses, and enlarge the sinus ostia to promote drainage.

Abbie returns to the office 1 week postoperatively for sinonasal debridement. She completes a course of postoperative steroids and antibiotics. Intraoperative cultures grew *Pseudomonas* and methicillin-resistant *Staphylococcus aureus* (MRSA). She then initiates culture-guided topical saline irrigations with compounded budesonide, tobramycin, and mupirocin twice daily. At 3 months postoperatively, Abbie notes significant improvement in symptoms with repeat SNOT-22 decreased to 20. Abbie continues to use medicated irrigations and follows up at 3-month intervals for surveillance, with significant improvement in her nasal endoscopy, seen in Fig. 9.2.

Conclusion

Rates of CRS approach 100% in patients with CF, although the degree of symptomatology varies. Comprehensive treatment of CF CRS includes a multidisciplinary team including a rhinologist. Therapy may include nasal saline irrigations and topical and/or systemic antibiotics, corticosteroids, and CFTR modulator therapy. Surgery is often indicated to improve gravity-dependent drainage and improve access to topical therapy. Appropriate management of CF CRS leads to an improvement in sinonasal symptoms, reduces pulmonary infections, and decreases inpatient hospitalization. Future research is necessary to further elucidate the effects of CRS on lower airway function and the optimal treatment strategy.

References

1. Rey MM, Bonk MP, Hadjiliadis D. Cystic fibrosis: emerging understanding and therapies. Annu Rev Med. 2019;70:197–210.
2. Tipirneni KE, Woodworth BA. Medical and surgical advancements in the management of cystic fibrosis chronic rhinosinusitis. Curr Otorhinolaryngol Rep. 2017;5:24–34.
3. Illing EA, Woodworth BA. Management of the upper airway in cystic fibrosis. Curr Opin Pulm Med. 2014;20:623–31.
4. Johansen HK, Aanaes K, Pressler T, Nielsen KG, Fisker J, Skov M, Høiby N, von Buchwald C. Colonisation and infection of the paranasal sinuses in cystic fibrosis patients is accompanied by a reduced PMN response. J Cyst Fibros. 2012;11:525–31.
5. Alanin MC, Aanaes K, Høiby N, Pressler T, Skov M, Nielsen KG, Taylor-Robinson D, Waldmann E, Krogh HJ. Sinus surgery postpones chronic gram-negative lung infection: cohort study of 106 patients with cystic fibrosis. Rhinology. 2016;54:206–13.
6. Orlandi RR, Kingdom TT, Hwang PH, Smith TL, Alt JA, Baroody FM, Batra PS, Bernal-Sprekelsen M, Bhattacharyya N, Chandra RK, et al. International consensus statement on allergy and rhinology: rhinosinusitis. Int Forum Allergy Rhinol. 2016;6:S22–S209.
7. Berkhout MC, Van Rooden CJ, Rijntjes E, Fokkens WJ, El Bouazzaoui LH, Heijerman HG. Sinonasal manifestations of cystic fibrosis: a correlation between genotype and phenotype? J Cyst Fibros. 2014;13:442–8.
8. Casserly P, Harrison M, O'Connell O, O'Donovan N, Plant BJ, O'Sullivan P. Nasal endoscopy and paranasal sinus computerised tomography (CT) findings in an Irish cystic fibrosis adult patient group. Eur Arch Otorhinolaryngol. 2015;272:3353–9.
9. Kang SH, Piltcher OB, de Tarso Roth Dalcin P. Sinonasal alterations in computed tomography scans in cystic fibrosis: a literature review of observational studies. Int Forum Allergy Rhinol. 2014;4:223–31.
10. Berkhout MC, Klerx-Melis F, Fokkens WJ, Nuijsink M, van Aalderen WM, Heijerman HG. CT-abnormalities, bacteriology and symptoms of sinonasal disease in children with cystic fibrosis. J Cyst Fibros. 2016;15:816–24.
11. Woodworth BA, Ahn C, Flume PA, Schlosser RJ. The delta F508 mutation in cystic fibrosis and impact on sinus development. Am J Rhinol. 2007;21:122–7.
12. Rasmussen J, Aanæs K, Norling R, Nielsen KG, Johansen HK, von Buchwald C. CT of the paranasal sinuses is not a valid indicator for sinus surgery in CF patients. J Cyst Fibros. 2012;11:93–9.
13. Habib AR, Quon BS, Buxton JA, Alsaleh S, Singer J, Manji J, Wicox PG, Javer AR. The Sino-Nasal Outcome Test–22 as a tool to identify chronic rhinosinusitis in adults with cystic fibrosis. Int Forum Allergy Rhinol. 2015;5:1111–7.
14. Habib AR, Buxton JA, Singer J, Wilcox PG, Javer AR, Quon BS. Association between chronic rhinosinusitis and health-related quality of life in adults with cystic fibrosis. Ann Am Thorac Soc. 2015;12:1163–9.
15. Mainz JG, Koitschev A. Management of chronic rhinosinusitis in CF. J Cyst Fibros. 2009;8:S10–4.
16. Cimmino M, Nardone M, Cavaliere M, Plantulli A, Sepe A, Esposito V, Mazzarella G, Raia V. Dornase alfa as postoperative therapy in cystic fibrosis sinonasal disease. Arch Otolaryngol Head Neck Surg. 2005;131:1097–101.

17. Mainz JG, Schien C, Schiller I, Schädlich K, Koitschev A, Koitschev C, Riethmüller J, Graepler-Mainka U, Wiedemann B, Beck JF. Sinonasal inhalation of dornase alfa administered by vibrating aerosol to cystic fibrosis patients: a double-blind placebo-controlled cross-over trial. J Cyst Fibros. 2014;13:461–70.
18. Mainz JG, Schumacher U, Schädlich K, Hentschel J, Koitschev C, Koitschev A, Riethmüller J, Prenzel F, Sommerburg O, Wiedemann B, et al. Sino nasal inhalation of isotonic versus hypertonic saline (6.0%) in CF patients with chronic rhinosinusitis—Results of a multicenter, prospective, randomized, double-blind, controlled trial. J Cyst Fibros. 2016;15:e57–66.
19. Aanaes K, Alanin MC, Nielsen KG, Møller MJ, Høiby N, Johansen HK, Johannesen HH, Mortensen J. The accessibility of topical treatment in the paranasal sinuses on operated cystic fibrosis patients assessed by scintigraphy. Rhinology. 2018;56:268–73.
20. Hadfield PJ, Rowe-Jones JM, Mackay IS. A prospective treatment trial of nasal polyps in adults with cystic fibrosis. Rhinology. 2000;38:63–5.
21. Donaldson JD, Gillespie CT. Observations on the efficacy of intranasal beclomethasone dipropionate in cystic fibrosis patients. J Otolaryngol. 1988;17:43–5.
22. Mainz JG, Schädlich K, Schien C, Michl R, Schelhorn-Neise P, Koitschev A, Koitschev C, Keller PM, Riethmüller J, Wiedemann B, et al. Sinonasal inhalation of tobramycin vibrating aerosol in cystic fibrosis patients with upper airway *Pseudomonas aeruginosa* colonization: results of a randomized, double-blind, placebo-controlled pilot study. Drug Des Dev Ther. 2014;8:209.
23. Moss RB, King VV. Management of sinusitis in cystic fibrosis by endoscopic surgery and serial antimicrobial lavage: reduction in recurrence requiring surgery. Arch Otolaryngol Head Neck Surg. 1995;121:566–72.
24. McCormick J, Cho DY, Lampkin B, Richman J, Hathorne H, Rowe SM, Woodworth BA. Ivacaftor improves rhinologic, psychologic, and sleep-related quality of life in G551D cystic fibrosis patients. Int Forum Allergy Rhinol. 2019;9:292–7.
25. Chang EH, Tang XX, Shah VS, Launspach JL, Ernst SE, Hilkin B, Karp PH, Abou Alaiwa MH, Graham SM, Hornick DB, et al. Medical reversal of chronic sinusitis in a cystic fibrosis patient with ivacaftor. Int Forum Allergy Rhinol. 2015;5:178–81.
26. Lindstrom DR, Conley SF, Splaingard ML, Gershan WM. Ibuprofen therapy and nasal polyposis in cystic fibrosis patients. J Otolaryngol. 2007;36:309–14.
27. Ayoub N, Thamboo A, Habib A-R, Nayak JV, Hwang PH. Determinants and outcomes of upfront surgery versus medical therapy for chronic rhinosinusitis in cystic fibrosis. Int Forum Allergy Rhinol. 2017;7(5):450–8.
28. Khalid AN, Mace J, Smith TL. Outcomes of sinus surgery in adults with cystic fibrosis. Otolaryngol Head Neck Surg. 2009;141(3):358–63.
29. MacDonald KI, Gipsman A, Magit A, et al. Endoscopic sinus surgery in patients with cystic fibrosis: a systematic review and meta-analysis of pulmonary function. Rhinology. 2012;50(4):360–9.
30. Liang J, Higgins TS, Ishman SL, Boss EF, Benke JR, Lin SY. Surgical management of chronic rhinosinusitis in cystic fibrosis: a systematic review. Int Forum Allergy Rhinol. 2013;3(10):814–22.
31. Eggesbø HB, Søvik S, Dølvik S, Eiklid K, Kolmannskog F. CT characterization of developmental variations of the paranasal sinuses in cystic fibrosis. Acta Radiol. 2001;42(5):482–93.
32. Do BAJ, Lands LC, Saint-Martin C, et al. Effect of the F508del genotype on outcomes of endoscopic sinus surgery in children with cystic fibrosis. Int J Pediatr Otorhinolaryngol. 2014;78(7):1133–7.
33. Rickert S, Banuchi VE, Germana JD, Stewart MG, April MM. Cystic fibrosis and endoscopic sinus surgery: relationship between nasal polyposis and likelihood of revision endoscopic sinus surgery in patients with cystic fibrosis. Arch Otolaryngol Head Neck Surg. 2010;136(10):988–92.
34. Jaberoo MC, Pulido MA, Saleh HA. Modified Lothrop procedure in cystic fibrosis patients: does it have a role? J Laryngol Otol. 2013;127(7):666–9.

35. Virgin FW, Rowe SM, Wade MB, et al. Extensive surgical and comprehensive postoperative medical management for cystic fibrosis chronic rhinosinusitis. Am J Rhinol Allergy. 2012;26(1):70–5.
36. Alanin MC, Aanaes K, Hoiby N, et al. Sinus surgery postpones chronic gram-negative lung infection: cohort study of 106 patients with cystic fibrosis. Rhinology J. 2017;54(3):206–13.
37. Aanaes K, von Buchwald C, Hjuler T, Skov M, Alanin M, Johansen HK. The effect of sinus surgery with intensive follow-up on pathogenic sinus bacteria in patients with cystic fibrosis. Am J Rhinol Allergy. 2013;27(1):e1–4.
38. Shatz A. Management of recurrent sinus disease in children with cystic fibrosis: a combined approach. Otolaryngol Head Neck Surg. 2006;135(2):248–52.
39. Rosbe KW, Jones DT, Rahbar R, Lahiri T, Auerbach AD. Endoscopic sinus surgery in cystic fibrosis: do patients benefit from surgery? Int J Pediatr Otorhinolaryngol. 2001;61(2):113–9.
40. Henriquez OA, Wolfenden LL, Stecenko A, DelGaudio JM, Wise SK. Endoscopic sinus surgery in adults with cystic fibrosis: effect on lung function, intravenous antibiotic use, and hospitalization. Arch Otolaryngol Head Neck Surg. 2012;138(12):1167–70.
41. Triglia JM, Nicollas R. Nasal and sinus polyposis in children. Laryngoscope. 1997;107(7): 963–6.
42. Kovell LC, Wang J, Ishman SL, Zeitlin PL, Boss EF. Cystic fibrosis and sinusitis in children: outcomes and socioeconomic status. Otolaryngol Head Neck Surg. 2011;145(1):146–53.
43. Holzmann D, Speich R, Kaufmann T, et al. Effects of sinus surgery in patients with cystic fibrosis after lung transplantation: a 10-year experience. Transplantation. 2004;77(1):134–6.
44. Vital D, Hofer M, Benden C, Holzmann D, Boehler A. Impact of sinus surgery on pseudomonal airway colonization, bronchiolitis obliterans syndrome and survival in cystic fibrosis lung transplant recipients. Respiration. 2013;86(1):25–31.

Chapter 10
Cystic Fibrosis and Chronic Rhinosinusitis: Interventions on the Horizon

Catherine Banks, Harrison Thompson, Jessica W. Grayson, Do-Yeon Cho, and Bradford A. Woodworth

Key Concepts
- Improved understanding of cystic fibrosis (CF) pathophysiology has led to significant recent advancements in CF therapeutics.
- Targeted mutation-specific modulators and potentiators have transformed CF care.
- The role of novel topical therapeutics and implants in the management of CF CRS is under active investigation.

C. Banks
Department of Otolaryngology-Head and Neck Surgery, Prince of Wales and Sydney Hospitals, University of New South Wales, Randwick, Sydney, NSW, Australia

H. Thompson · J. W. Grayson
Department of Otolaryngology Head and Neck Surgery, University of Alabama at Birmingham School of Medicine, Birmingham, AL, USA

D.-Y. Cho
Department of Otolaryngology Head and Neck Surgery, University of Alabama at Birmingham School of Medicine, Birmingham, AL, USA

Gregory Fleming James Cystic Fibrosis Research Center, Birmingham, AL, USA

B. A. Woodworth (✉)
Gregory Fleming James Cystic Fibrosis Research Center, Birmingham, AL, USA

Department of Otolaryngology-Head and Neck Surgery, University of Alabama at Birmingham, Birmingham, AL, USA
e-mail: bwoodworth@uabmc.edu

© Springer Nature Switzerland AG 2020
D. A. Gudis, R. J. Schlosser (eds.), *The Unified Airway*,
https://doi.org/10.1007/978-3-030-50330-7_10

Introduction

Thirty years ago, identification and sequencing of the cystic fibrosis (CF) gene provided the foundation to understand CF pathogenesis and drove the development of the therapeutic options now available to patients [1, 2]. Recent knowledge regarding the pathophysiology of CF pulmonary and sinonasal disease has led to changes to treatment strategies and improved morbidity and mortality. Thus, an up-to-date understanding of the underlying pathogenic mechanisms and therapeutic modalities available is necessary for the modern clinician to provide the most effective care for their patients.

Definition/Description of the Disorder

CF is an autosomal recessive genetic disorder caused by a mutation of the gene encoding the CF transmembrane conductance regulator (CFTR) protein [3]. CF has broad implications in the nasal cavity, paranasal sinuses, and pulmonary and digestive systems with downstream consequences, including diabetes, protein and nutrient malabsorption, male infertility, and increased susceptibility to airway bacterial infections due to impaired mucociliary clearance (MCC) [3, 4].

Epidemiology and Incidence

The highest incidence of CF is reported in the European population (ranging between 1:2000 and 1:3000 live births), and the lowest incidence is in Asian populations (ranging between 1:40,000 and 1:100,000 live births) [1]. Due to ethnic heterogeneity, the United States has approximately 30,000 individuals who carry the diagnosis of CF with an incidence of roughly 1 in every 3500 live births [5, 6].

Demographic characteristics are important when considering the gene variation among these populations. While northern European patients are most likely to exhibit the most common CF mutation (F508del), other populations may display differing genetic profiles, which may delay diagnosis, worsen outcomes, and reduce access to critical treatment modalities [7, 8].

Advancements in treatment have led to an increase in life expectancy, with half of the individuals born from 2014 to 2018 now predicted to live beyond 44.4 years of age [9].

Etiology and Pathogenesis

CF is caused by a mutation of the q31 locus of the long arm of chromosome 7 that encodes for the CF transmembrane conductance regulator (CFTR) protein [3]. The protein channel in unaffected individuals is present and functional at the apical

Table 10.1 Classification of CFTR mutations

Class	Mutation example	Cellular/molecular phenotype
I	W1282X	Absent CFTR production due to nonsense mutations, frameshift mutations, or abnormal mRNA splicing
II	ΔF508	Improper intracellular processing of CFTR with less than normal amounts of CFTR protein at the apical plasma membrane
III	G551D	Defective regulation of CFTR channels at the apical plasma membrane
IV	R117H	Defective permeation of anions through CFTR channels at the apical plasma membrane
V	3849+10KbC>T	Reduced synthesis of normal CFTR
VI	Q1412X	Altered apical membrane residence time of CFTR channels with truncated c-terminus

Adapted (with permission pending) from Kreindler [10]

surface of epithelial cells, where it primarily functions as a chloride (Cl⁻) and bicarbonate (HCO_3^-) channel to regulate hydration and viscosity of the airway surface liquid (ASL). There are over 1700 mutations identified in the CFTR, and they are classified according to 6 categories (Table 10.1) [10]. The first three classes (I-III) are associated with increased severity. Class I mutations occur due to an absence of CFTR gene synthesis and develop secondary to premature termination codons, nonsense mutations, (e.g., G542X) or other out-of-frame mutations (insertions or deletions). In class II mutations, the CFTR is normally transcribed or translated; however, the protein folds incorrectly and is recognized as defective in the endoplasmic reticulum and degraded before it reaches its site of action at the cell surface. The F508del mutation (deletion of a phenylalanine residual at the 508 position) is the most common genetic mutation and accounts for approximately 70% of defective alleles. Class III mutations consist of full-length CFTR protein present in normal quantities at the cell surface, yet regulation or gating of the Cl⁻ transporter is disrupted, which causes reduced ion channel activity (e.g., G551D). Class IV defects have partial activity in vivo, resulting in phenotypes that can be less severe (e.g., R117H mutation). Class V mutations represent decreased quantities of CFTR transcripts and fewer functional CFTR channels at the cell surface. Class VI mutations create defects in the stability of the protein, leading to increased turnover at the cell surface and therefore reduced quantities of CFTR under steady-state conditions [6]. When CFTR dysfunction is present, reduced ion transport leads to improper hydration, and thickening of the ASL with viscosity increased up to 30–60 times that of non-CF patients [11]. This highly tenacious mucous reduces MCC, obstructing sinus ostia and creating a hypoxic environment with subsequent mucosal edema, ciliary dyskinesia, and bacterial overgrowth leading to CRS.

CRS incidence approaches almost 100% in CF patients. It not only is a common cause of morbidity but also worsens pulmonary outcomes and mortality [4, 11–14]. CF patients exhibit similar bacterial colonization of the paranasal sinuses compared to the lower respiratory tract, suggesting that the sinonasal cavities serve as a reservoir for pathogens that exacerbate pulmonary symptoms and reinfections [13–15]. Additionally, colonization with biofilm-forming organisms (e.g., *P. aeruginosa* in the upper airway) is believed to be a key pathogenic factor in lower respiratory tract disease via direct seeding of organisms [1, 4, 16–21]. The surgical management of sinus disease in CF patients has been demonstrated to lead to reduced hospitalization and symptom burden, indicating that alleviating sinonasal disease has implications beyond QoL [4, 16, 17].

Clinical Presentation

Sixty-four percent of patients with CF in the United States are diagnosed at infancy while asymptomatic or minimally symptomatic due to government-mandated newborn screening. These screening tools rely on the detection of high levels of trypsinogen levels in the newborn's blood due to abnormal drainage and recycling of the pancreatic enzyme into the gastrointestinal tract [22, 23]. Positive screening is typically followed by a genetic screen or sweat chloride test with levels greater than or equal to 60 mmol/L being diagnostic for CF [24]. Despite advances in early diagnosis, over one-third of CF patients are not diagnosed by newborn screening. Therefore, the practicing clinician must be suspicious of CF as a possibility when recurrent sinopulmonary infections and other CF sequelae are present, regardless of previous newborn screening results.

The typical presentation of CF includes a multiorgan system symptomatology including, but not limited to, recurrent upper and lower respiratory infection, CRS, pancreatic insufficiency, meconium ileus, and infertility. While most CF diagnoses are made in childhood, there is growing recognition of less common phenotypes that are identified at older ages that still cause considerable morbidity. Respiratory illness, gastrointestinal complaints, and sinonasal disease with or without nasal polyposis are the most common symptoms that lead to diagnosis in adulthood [25, 26].

Sinonasal Findings in CF

Endoscopic findings include local inflammation, purulent drainage, and the presence of nasal polyps with or without nasal obstruction. Nasal polyposis is found in 10%–32% of patients with CF with a gross anatomic structure similar to that observed in allergic or eosinophilic polyposis. However, on histopathology, there is a relative neutrophilic predominance in CF patients [11, 27–29].

Radiographic Findings in CF

Radiographic findings in CF will vary depending on the clinical course and genetic profile of the patient, with homozygous F508del patients particularly affected [30–32]. The vast majority of patients (90%–100%) will show near-complete opacification of the sinuses on computed tomography (CT) imaging by 8 months of age [27].

Varying degrees of sinus developmental abnormalities are present, including hypo-plasia (especially in the frontal and sphenoid sinuses), lateral nasal wall erosion, and uncinate demineralization [31–33]. CT may reveal medialization of the lateral nasal wall due to the presence of pseudomucoceles, a structure of multiloculated collec-tions of pus surrounded by a thickened mucosal lining. These are typically found bilaterally and in the maxillary sinus in children under 5 years of age [31, 34]. Despite these common findings, routine CT scanning is not recommended in patients unless symptomatic or abnormalities on endoscopy are noted [35, 36].

Medical Management and Outcomes

Medical treatment remains the initial management for CF CRS. While there are consensus guidelines for the treatment of non-CF CRS [21, 37], there are no univer-sally accepted guidelines for the management of the CF CRS population [17]. Although the data is sparse and heterogeneous, there are several recent studies that demonstrate favorable outcomes with medical management in CF CRS [38–40].

Systemic Medical Therapy

Systemic Corticosteroids

Systemic corticosteroids and antibiotics remain the most frequent medications used by otolaryngologists; however, there is a lack of long-term specific CF outcome data showing significant benefit for these medications [41]. Non-CF patients with nasal polyps receive benefit from a short course (2–4 weeks) of oral corticosteroids [42], yet the use of short-term treatment in CF patients remains controversial. A recent survey involving the members of the American Society of Pediatric Otolaryngology (ASPO) and the American Rhinology Society (ARS) revealed that 57.9% of pediat-ric otolaryngologists would use oral steroids in CF CRS [19].

CF CRS is predominately a neutrophilic driven inflammatory response, and neu-trophils have been shown to be less responsive to steroids than eosinophils [43]. To date, no study has investigated the use of systemic steroids for CF CRS. Caution is warranted with the use of systemic corticosteroids as the adverse events associated with corticosteroid use in the CF population, such as increased blood sugar, are further complicated by CF-related pancreatic dysfunction [44].

Systemic Antibiotics

Chronic airway infection secondary to opportunistic bacterial colonization with *P. aeruginosa* and *Staphylococcus aureus* are common afflictions in CF-CRS patients, and antibiotic therapy should typically be directed at these common pathogens with culture-directed treatment [43]. Numerous bacteria isolated from sinus culture studies reinforce the role of the sinonasal cavities as a reservoir for pathogens that exacerbate pulmonary symptoms [13–15, 45]. However, unlike the role of antibiotics for respiratory exacerbations in CF, there is a paucity of literature on the role of systemic antibiotics in CF CRS. Lowery et al. [19] showed that 85.1% of pediatric otolaryngologists advocate for the use of oral antibiotics and 40.4% support the use of intravenous antibiotics in CF CRS management. Aanaes et al. [46] demonstrated that the use of intensive antibiotic therapy was beneficial during the postoperative period in the eradication of chronic sinonasal bacterial colonization [46]. This study showed two-thirds of patients had no pathogenic bacteria from cultures taken from the maxillary-ethmoidal complex for 6 months post-ESS following a 2-week regime of broad-spectrum intravenous antibiotics, 6 months of colistin nasal irrigations, and 12 months of topical nasal steroids [46].

Macrolide antibiotics are beneficial for their anti-inflammatory properties [47]. Commonly used macrolides such as azithromycin and clarithromycin promote tissue repair by modulating the inflammatory response by inciting reduced neutrophil chemotaxis, decreasing mucus production and cytokine release, and improving the clearance of airway secretions [43]. Clinically, patients see reduced nasal secretions, postnasal drainage, and improvements in nasal obstruction [48].

CFTR Modulators

Advanced genetic research has opened the door for novel therapies targeting the basic defect in the CFTR protein. Restoration of function to apical anion secretion is possible due to drugs that target the dysfunctional protein rather than the consequences of the disease. Two classes of CFTR modulators are currently available and Food and Drug Administration (FDA) approved for the treatment of patients with CF: (1) correctors, which increase defective CFTR protein processing and trafficking to the cell surface, and (2) potentiators, which improve mutant CFTR protein activity (channel opening/open probability) at the cell surface [49]. Correctors and potentiators are also used in combination to enhance CFTR activity [49].

Ivacaftor (Kalydeco [VX-770], Vertex pharmaceuticals Inc.) is a CFTR potentiator that improves the open probability of the defective Cl$^-$ channel in patients with at least one copy of the mutant G551D-CFTR allele or other less common loss-of-function mutations affecting gating (non-G551D class III and residual function mutations) [50–52]. The role of ivacaftor treatment in pulmonary CF is well documented with significant improvements observed in lung function. A multicenter prospective cohort study also identified significant improvements in QoL via the sinonasal outcome test-20 (SNOT-20) at 1 month, 3 months, and 6 months posttreatment with ivacaftor, with improvement observed within the rhinologic, physiological, and sleep domains of the SNOT-20 [53].

The next therapeutic approach was to combine a CFTR corrector of F508del CFTR (permits processing of the protein such that a percentage will be transported to the apical membrane) with CFTR potentiators. Lumacaftor/ivacaftor (Orkambi ™ [VX-809] Vertex pharmaceutical Inc.) was initially FDA approved to treat patients 12 years and older homozygous for the F508del mutation. This combination drug conferred improvements in forced expiratory volume in 1 second (FEV1), reduced pulmonary exacerbations, and enabled a 40% reduction in the yearly rate of pulmonary deterioration. Subsequent approval of the corrector tezacaftor (VX-659) with ivacaftor (SymdekoTM, Vertex Pharmaceuticals Inc.) provided similar benefits but with decreased incidence of side effects (e.g., chest tightness) [54]. Unfortunately, neither combination of corrector (either lumacaftor or tezacaftor) with a potentiator (ivacaftor) showed efficacy in patients heterozygous for F508del CFTR coupled with a minimal function mutation (mutation associated with no protein production or *no* in vitro response to ivacaftor or ivacaftor/tezacaftor) [55]. While the respiratory symptoms were not significantly improved, an increase in body mass index, which is often reduced in CF patients, was noted, suggesting improved gastrointestinal health [20, 56].

Because tezacaftor and lumacaftor correct only approximately 15% of the protein [57, 58], a strategy to improve the efficiency of correction by increasing the quantity of apical membrane protein using two correctors together was attempted to improve clinical benefit. Elexacaftor/ivacaftor/tezacaftor (Trikafta™ [VX-445] Vertex Pharmaceutical Inc.) received its first approval in the United States in October 2019 for the treatment of CF in patients aged ≥ 12 years who have ≥ 1 F508del mutation in the *CFTR* gene [59]. It is the first triple combination therapy to treat patients with the most common CF mutation. Clinical impact was very robust with average improvement in lung function (FEV1) of 14.8%.

The efficacy of CFTR modulators in the lower airway is well established. While there is only a single study on CF CRS and CFTR modulators [53] showing improved sinus-related QoL, the premise of the unified airway theory supports their use for CF CRS in this advancing field. Because CFTR modulators impact CFTR function, their utility in other diseases of mucus clearance and acquired CFTR dysfunction such as COPD and CRS also shows promise as a therapeutic approach [60–73].

Future Directions: Systemic Genetic Therapies

Novel technologies have generated new approaches to genetic therapies, especially in relation to CFTR mRNA therapy and CRISPR gene editing (with the possibility of editing progenitor cells). CFTR mRNA is one of the most promising new therapies on the horizon for CF patients. This therapy is an alternative approach to correct or replace the abnormal mRNA transcribed by mutant CFTR genes. The approach uses lipid nanoparticles to deliver CFTR mRNA to the airway epithelium by inhalation [74, 75]. The delivery of normal CFTR complementary DNA suggests that all CF patients may benefit irrespective of the underlying CFTR variants. Phase I and II clinical trials have been encouraging. (TranslateBio) [76] The CRISPR (clustered regularly interspaced palindromic repeats)-Cas9 (CRISPR-Associated) nuclease is an editing system designed to target genes for correcting or modulating their expression [77]. The mechanism relies on two components: the RNA guide which acts as a custodian and a Cas protein complex which functions as a highly precise molecular knife. The guide RNA can be altered to match the DNA sequence of interest in the cell and accordingly be used to rectify mutations that may otherwise cause disease [78]. However, these rapidly developing technologies are still at their infancy because delivery of sufficient quantities and durable, sufficient expression persistence at disease sites remains elusive [76].

Topical Medical Therapy

Nasal Saline Irrigations

Intranasal saline irrigations act as a lavage and mechanically debride the sinonasal cavities to remove the viscous mucus and inflammatory mediators that impair clearance of debris and bacteria. Although saline irrigations are the basis of CRS management, there is no study to date that has evaluated efficacy in a CF CRS cohort. A recent Cochrane meta-analysis concluded that the use of isotonic saline (0.9%) irrigation in the non-CF population resulted in symptomatic improvement and amelioration of disease-specific QOL outcomes when compared to no treatment [79, 80]. Hypertonic saline provides the additional benefit of creating an osmotic gradient and hydration of mucus to decrease its viscosity. It is also suggested that the mucosa decongests because water is drawn from the inflamed mucosa to the airway surface [31]. However, a double-blind, crossover randomized control trial comparing nebulized hypertonic 6.0% saline versus isotonic 0.9% saline in CF CRS patients showed that hypertonic saline did not exhibit any benefit over 0.9% saline according to SNOT-20 score at 28 days [81]. Hypertonic saline irrigations may also be poorly tolerated in patients due to nasal irritation, which could impact patient compliance.

Corticosteroids

Intranasal corticosteroids (INCS) are known to be efficacious in CRS; yet, the effect in CF is less clear [82]. Tran et al. identified only one study assessing INCS in CF CRS [83]. This study compared intranasal betamethasone drops twice daily to placebo and found that there was no symptomatic difference at 6 weeks between the two groups, despite endoscopic Lund-McKay scores showing a decrease in polyp size [84]. Interestingly, low-absorption topical steroid rinses (i.e., mometasone and budesonide) are routinely prescribed for both CF and non-CF-related CRS given the anti-inflammatory properties and low side-effect profile [4]. Budesonide has not been shown to produce any significant effect on the hypothalamic-pituitary axis [85–87].

Antibiotics

Topical antibiotics are a key component of CF CRS therapy. The benefit of topical antibiotics over systemic antibiotics is the higher local concentration in the sinuses with a low risk of antibiotic systemic side effects. Mainz et al. undertook a double-blind, randomized placebo-controlled study of intranasal tobramycin in six CF patients with sinonasal colonization of *P. aeruginosa*. In this study, nebulized vibrating sinonasal tobramycin (80 mg/2 ml) was delivered in an aerosol form for 4 minutes per nostril over a period of 28 days and showed significantly improved SNOT-20 scores ($p = 0.033$) and reduced *Pseudomonas* colonization in 67% of treated patients compared to 3 (50%) in the placebo group; however, this difference was not statistically significant [39]. Another retrospective study showed that post-operative topical aminoglycoside with nasal irrigation resulted in reduced recurrence of CF-related sinus exacerbations and infection due to *P. aeruginosa* as well as improved control of CRS for up to 2 years [88].

Dornase Alfa

Dornase alfa is a mucolytic agent that is derived from recombinant deoxyribonuclease. It functions by cleaving extracellular long-chain DNA, which accumulates in CF airways as a result of extensive neutrophil degradation and serves as a dominant contributor to the viscosity of CF mucus and sputum [43]. A systematic review assessed the efficacy of nebulized dornase alfa in 104 patients across 6 studies [89]. Four studies used standardized nebulizers via facemask or nasal adapter, and two studies used a pulsating aerosolizer. All six studies showed improvement in patient symptom scores regardless of the delivery device, although the impact on radiology, endoscopy, and pulmonary function outcomes was variable across studies.

Drug-Eluting Sinus Stents

Steroid-eluting sinus stents were developed to improve postsurgical healing and complications, reduce the need for revision surgery, and mitigate issues with patient adherence or compliance. Placement of steroid-eluting sinus stents after ESS has been shown to reduce polyp development, adhesion formation, and future interventions. Additionally, steroid-eluting sinus stents are a more cost-effective intervention than traditional postsurgical management [90, 91]. However, CF patients were excluded from all studies related to this device.

Recently, antibiotic-eluting sinus stents have emerged as a potential therapeutic approach to treat biofilm-related chronic sinus infections, which are predominant in CF sinuses. Stents are composed of poly-D/L-lactic acid (PLLA), a mesh material that can appropriately expand and conform to the shape of the sinus cavity. Additionally, these stents can be coated with poly (D, L-lactide-co-glycolide) (PLGA) nanoparticles to allow loading of a drug of choice onto the exterior of the matrix. Steroid-eluting stents were previously approved by the FDA in 2010, making the creation of antibiotic-eluting stents ideal for further therapeutic development [92, 93].

Cho et al. [94] created a ciprofloxacin-eluting sinus stent (CSS) that demonstrated efficacy against *Pseudomonas* biofilms in vitro and in an in vivo clinical model of rabbit *Pseudomonas* sinusitis. The local release of ciprofloxacin to the sinus mucosa permits high concentrations of antibiotic delivery without systemic exposure that is present in oral or intravenous treatment. Unfortunately, the pharmacokinetic profile of the CSS revealed a burst-release phenomenon that did not supply sustained concentrations of ciprofloxacin during the study period, likely due to the hydrophilic nature of ciprofloxacin. For this reason, the ciprofloxacin-ivacaftor sinus stent (CISS) was developed, which advanced the initial concept of the CSS by adding a second, hydrophobic layer of the CFTR potentiator, ivacaftor, incorporated in nanoparticles. This successfully stifled the burst-release phenomenon observed in the CSS studies while also allowing sustained controlled release of ivacaftor and ciprofloxacin to the sinus mucosa for 3 weeks [94–96].

In addition to improving the antibiotic release profile, ivacaftor provides additional therapeutic benefits due to its role as a CFTR potentiator. The CISS demonstrated improvements in rabbit sinus potential difference indicating improved CFTR function and mucociliary clearance. Additionally, ivacaftor potentiates the antibacterial properties of ciprofloxacin to improve efficacy against pseudomonal biofilms [96–98].

Surgical Management and Outcomes

Surgical Approach

There is no current consensus guideline for when to offer endoscopic sinus surgery (ESS) to patients with CF CRS, but surgery is a critical therapeutic option for CF CRS refractory to medical therapy. Studies have shown that 20%–60% of CF patients eventually require surgery [20, 46, 99]. ESS offers both symptomatic, radiographic, and endoscopic improvement [100]. Systematic reviews have demonstrated a QoL benefit in CF CRS patients undergoing ESS. However, there is a lack of high-level evidence supporting surgical management [101, 102]. In non-CF CRS, ESS focuses on opening obstructed sinus ostia and allowing improved sinonasal drainage and permitting adequate penetration of topical medications [43]. In CF CRS, a more extensive surgical modification of the maxillary sinus has been advocated in a number of studies due to high revision ESS rates and to facilitate easier debridement of the sinonasal cavities in the clinical setting [103–105]. The maxillary sinus remains a recurrent problem in CF patients due to its superiorly located ostia and accumulation of mucopurulence within. The MEMM demonstrated significant improvement in the effectiveness of nasal irrigations and delivery of topical treatments and permitted improved access for debridement in the clinic. Improved symptom scores using SNOT-22 questionnaires (64.7 ± 18.4 presurgery versus 27.5 ± 15.3 postsurgery; $p < 0.0001$), at 60 days, remained decreased through to 1 year postoperatively (27.6 ± 12.6; $p < 0.0001$), and significantly reduced Lund-Kennedy endoscopy scores (10.4 ± 1.1 presurgery versus 5.7 ± 1.4 postsurgery at

60 days; $p < 0.0001$) and 6.0 ± 1.1; $p < 0.0001$) were observed up to 12 months post-op [106]. Although FEV1 did not improve at 1-year postoperatively, the mean number of pulmonary-related hospitalizations did significantly decrease in the first postoperative year compared to the previous year before surgery. These results were supported by an earlier study in children, where there was significant improvement in QoL, reduced need for IV antibiotics, and decreased rate of inpatient hospitalizations [107]. This study also found a significant improvement in FEV1 at 6 months [107]. Similarly, Khalfoun et al. [108] performed a retrospective review in 2018 of 181 CF patients with moderate to severe lung disease and found postoperative improvement across multiple PFT metrics at 1 year following ESS [108]. However, a systematic review did not identify improvement in PFT scores [101]. Of the eight studies (level 3b to level 4) that examined PFT outcomes as a measure for the effectiveness of surgical therapy [106, 107, 109–114], only one [111] (level 3b evidence) showed improvements in PFT scores. Furthermore, ESS in CF CRS patients who have undergone lung transplantation does not appear to improve PFTs [115, 116]. Leung et al. [116] demonstrated that sinus surgery before bilateral lung transplant does not appear to prevent lung graft recolonization and is not associated with an overall survival benefit, although there were several limitations in this study.

Impact of Rhinologic Interventions on Medical Disorder

Medical and surgical interventions play critical roles in the management of CF CRS. Although there is no high-level evidence to recommend a "gold standard" approach in CF patients, the role of multimodality and multidisciplinary approaches is essential. Evidence supports the use of topical antibiotics, DNAse mucolytics, and CFTR modulators. However, support for corticosteroids and systemic antibiotics is lacking. Surgery including both standard ESS and extended surgical approaches improve sinonasal outcomes, yet the benefit with respect to pulmonary outcomes remains less clear.

Case Presentations

Case 1

A 30-year-old male with CF CRS (F508del/1154insTC) initially presented at age 22 years with a history of six prior endoscopic sinus surgeries. He had symptomatic CRS with evidence of pansinusitis (Fig. 10.1). He underwent bilateral FESS with MEMM with improved sustained control of the lower sinuses with chronic corticosteroid and tobramycin irrigation. However, his frontal sinus continued to have polypoid edema and frequent flare-ups (Fig. 10.2a).

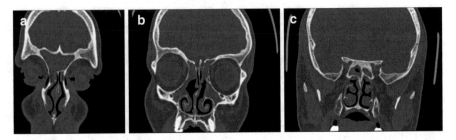

Fig. 10.1 Coronal CT images depicting pansinus opacification despite previous surgical interventions. Hypoplastic frontal, maxillary, and sphenoid sinuses are present

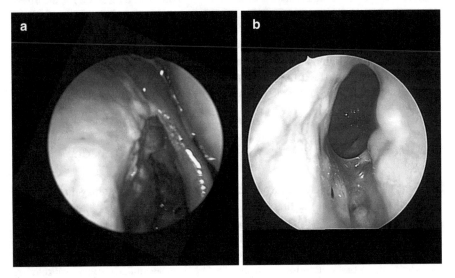

Fig. 10.2 Endoscopic images of the right frontal sinus. (**a**) Polypoid edema, bacterial colonization, and overall poor mucosal control. (**b**) Right frontal sinus widely patent without bacterial colonization or polypoid recurrence following initiation of CFTR modulators (Trikafta)

He was recently placed on Trikafta with vast improvement in control of his frontal sinus disease (Fig. 10.2b).

Case 2

A 31-year-old female with a history of CF CRS (F508del homozygous) initially presented with poor nasal breathing, facial pain and pressure, and hyposmia. She had multiple previous sinus surgeries with persistent radiographic and clinical disease. Her nasal endoscopy revealed a lateralized left middle turbinate. She had minimal polypoid edema on the left and mucopurulence present on the right (Fig. 10.3).

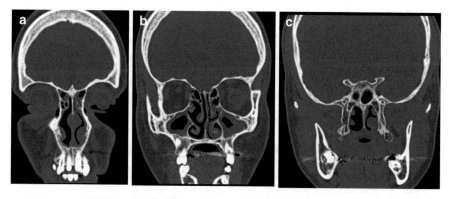

Fig. 10.3 Coronal CT images depicting pansinus mucosal thickening following previous surgeries

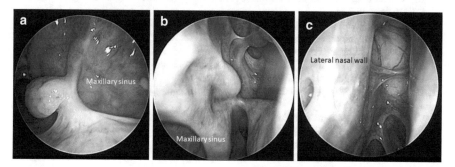

Fig. 10.4 Endoscopy images following endoscopic sinus surgery with modified endoscopic medial maxillectomies and routine use of topical corticosteroid and antibiotic rinses

She underwent revision bilateral FESS with MEMM in 2010. Following surgery, she has had well-controlled sinuses with chronic topical tobramycin and corticosteroid saline irrigations for 10 years (Fig. 10.4a–c).

Conclusion

The management of CF CRS remains a challenge to the otolaryngologist. A multidisciplinary collaboration and awareness of both the medical and surgical modalities are necessary for the modern clinician to provide the most effective care for patients. Despite the lack of high-level evidence available, evolving evidence supports the use of topical antibiotics, DNAse mucolytics, CFTR modulators, and ESS in the management of CRS for CF patients. Antibiotic-eluting sinus stents are in the treatment pipeline and may serve as an additional therapy for biofilm-forming infections in CF CRS.

Disclosures   Bradford A. Woodworth, MD, is a consultant for Cook Medical, Smith and Nephew, and Baxter.

References

1. Karanth TK, Karanth VKLK, Ward BK, Woodworth BA, Karanth L. Medical interventions for chronic rhinosinusitis in cystic fibrosis. Cochrane Database Syst Rev. 2019;10:CD012979.
2. Riordan JR, Rommens JM, Kerem B, Alon N, Rozmahel R, Grzelczak Z, et al. Identification of the cystic fibrosis gene: cloning and characterization of complementary DNA. Science. 1989;245(4922):1066–73.
3. Collins FS. Cystic fibrosis: molecular biology and therapeutic implications. Science. 1992;256(5058):774–9.
4. Illing EA, Woodworth BA. Management of the upper airway in cystic fibrosis. Curr Opin Pulm Med. 2014;20(6):623–31.
5. Corriveau S, Sykes J, Stephenson AL. Cystic fibrosis survival: the changing epidemiology. Curr Opin Pulm Med. 2018;24(6):574–8.
6. Rowe SM, Miller S, Sorscher EJ. Cystic fibrosis. N Engl J Med. 2005;352(19):1992–2001.
7. Bobadilla JL, Macek M Jr, Fine JP, Farrell PM. Cystic fibrosis: a worldwide analysis of CFTR mutations--correlation with incidence data and application to screening. Hum Mutat. 2002;19(6):575–606.
8. Elborn JS. Cystic fibrosis. Lancet (London, England). 2016;388(10059):2519–31.
9. Cystic Fibrosis Foundation Patient Registry. 2018 Annual data report. Bethesda, Maryland. ©2019 Cystic Fibrosis Foundation.
10. Kreindler JL. Cystic fibrosis: exploiting its genetic basis in the hunt for new therapies. Pharmacol Ther. 2010;125(2):219–29.
11. Gentile VG, Isaacson G. Patterns of sinusitis in cystic fibrosis. Laryngoscope. 1996;106(8):1005–9.
12. Chang EH. New insights into the pathogenesis of cystic fibrosis sinusitis. Int Forum Allergy Rhinol. 2014;4(2):132–7.
13. Choi KJ, Cheng TZ, Honeybrook AL, Gray AL, Snyder LD, Palmer SM, et al. Correlation between sinus and lung cultures in lung transplant patients with cystic fibrosis. Int Forum Allergy Rhinol. 2018;8(3):389–93.
14. Pletcher SD, Goldberg AN, Cope EK. Loss of microbial niche specificity between the upper and lower airways in patients with cystic fibrosis. Laryngoscope. 2019;129(3):544–50.
15. Morlacchi LC, Greer M, Tudorache I, Blasi F, Welte T, Haverich A, et al. The burden of sinus disease in cystic fibrosis lung transplant recipients. Transpl Infect Dis. 2018;20(5):e12924.
16. Hoiby N, Bjarnsholt T, Moser C, Jensen PO, Kolpen M, Qvist T, et al. Diagnosis of biofilm infections in cystic fibrosis patients. APMIS. 2017;125(4):339–43.
17. Gysin C, Alothman GA, Papsin BC. Sinonasal disease in cystic fibrosis: clinical characteristics, diagnosis, and management. Pediatr Pulmonol. 2000;30(6):481–9.
18. Chaaban MR, Kejner A, Rowe SM, Woodworth BA. Cystic fibrosis chronic rhinosinusitis: a comprehensive review. Am J Rhinol Allergy. 2013;27(5):387–95.
19. Lowery AS, Gallant JN, Woodworth BA, Brown RF, Sawicki GS, Shannon CN, et al. Chronic rhino-sinusitis treatment in children with cystic fibrosis: a cross-sectional survey of pediatric pulmonologists and otolaryngologists. Int J Pediatr Otorhinolaryngol. 2019;124:139–42.
20. Tipirneni KE, Woodworth BA. Medical and surgical advancements in the management of cystic fibrosis chronic rhinosinusitis. Curr Otorhinolaryngol Rep. 2017;5(1):24–34.
21. Orlandi RR, Kingdom TT, Hwang PH, Smith TL, Alt JA, Baroody FM, et al. International consensus statement on allergy and rhinology: rhinosinusitis. Int Forum Allergy Rhinol. 2016;6(Suppl 1):S22–209.
22. Castellani C, Massie J, Sontag M, Southern KW. Newborn screening for cystic fibrosis. Lancet Respir Med. 2016;4(8):653–61.
23. Farrell PM, White TB, Howenstine MS, Munck A, Parad RB, Rosenfeld M, et al. Diagnosis of cystic fibrosis in screened populations. J Pediatr. 2017;181S:S33–S44.e2.
24. Farrell PM, White TB, Ren CL, Hempstead SE, Accurso F, Derichs N, et al. Diagnosis of cystic fibrosis: consensus guidelines from the cystic fibrosis foundation. J Pediatr. 2017;181S:S4–S15.e1.

25. Sosnay PR, White TB, Farrell PM, Ren CL, Derichs N, Howenstine MS, et al. Diagnosis of cystic fibrosis in nonscreened populations. J Pediatr. 2017;181S:S52–S7.e2.
26. Keating CL, Liu X, Dimango EA. Classic respiratory disease but atypical diagnostic testing distinguishes adult presentation of cystic fibrosis. Chest. 2010;137(5):1157–63.
27. Ramsey B, Richardson MA. Impact of sinusitis in cystic fibrosis. J Allergy Clin Immunol. 1992;90(3 Pt 2):547–52.
28. Yung MW, Gould J, Upton GJG. Nasal polyposis in children with cystic fibrosis: a long-term follow-up study. Ann Otol Rhinol Laryngol. 2002;111(12 Pt 1):1081–6.
29. Hamilos DL. Chronic rhinosinusitis in patients with cystic fibrosis. J Allergy Clin Immunol Pract. 2016;4(4):605–12.
30. Woodworth BA, Ahn C, Flume PA, Schlosser RJ. The delta F508 mutation in cystic fibrosis and impact on sinus development. Am J Rhinol. 2007;21(1):122–7.
31. Kang SH, Dalcin PTR, Piltcher OB, Migliavacca RO. Chronic rhinosinusitis and nasal polyposis in cystic fibrosis: update on diagnosis and treatment. J Bras Pneumol. 2015;41(1):65–76.
32. Halderman AA, Lee S, London NR, Day A, Jain R, Moore JA, et al. Impact of high- versus low-risk genotype on sinonasal radiographic disease in cystic fibrosis. Laryngoscope. 2019;129(4):788–93.
33. April MA. CT scan findings of the paranasal sinuses in cystic fibrosis. Am J Rhinol. 1995;9:277–80.
34. Brihaye P, Jorissen M, Clement PA. Chronic rhinosinusitis in cystic fibrosis (mucoviscidosis). Acta Otorhinolaryngol Belg. 1997;51(4):323–37.
35. Gergin O, Kawai K, MacDougall RD, Robson CD, Moritz E, Cunningham M, et al. Sinus computed tomography imaging in pediatric cystic fibrosis: added value? Otolaryngol Head Neck Surg. 2016;155(1):160–5.
36. O'Connell OJ, McWilliams S, McGarrigle A, O'Connor OJ, Shanahan F, Mullane D, et al. Radiologic imaging in cystic fibrosis: cumulative effective dose and changing trends over 2 decades. Chest. 2012;141(6):1575–83.
37. Fokkens WJ, Lund VJ, Hopkins C, Hellings PW, Kern R, Reitsma S, et al. European position paper on rhinosinusitis and nasal polyps 2020. Rhinology. 2020;58(Suppl S29):1–464.
38. Mainz JG, Schien C, Schiller I, Schädlich K, Koitschev A, Koitschev C, et al. Sinonasal inhalation of dornase alfa administered by vibrating aerosol to cystic fibrosis patients: a double-blind placebo-controlled cross-over trial. J Cyst Fibros. 2014;13(4):461–70.
39. Mainz JG, Schädlich K, Schien C, Michl R, Schelhorn-Neise P, Koitschev A, et al. Sinonasal inhalation of tobramycin vibrating aerosol in cystic fibrosis patients with upper airway Pseudomonas aeruginosa colonization: results of a randomized, double-blind, placebo-controlled pilot study. Drug Des Devel Ther. 2014;8:209–17.
40. O'Connor MG, Seegmiller A. The effects of ivacaftor on CF fatty acid metabolism: an analysis from the GOAL study. J Cyst Fibros. 2017;16(1):132–8.
41. Chang MT, Patel ZM. Update on long-term outcomes for chronic rhinosinusitis in cystic fibrosis. Curr Opin Otolaryngol Head Neck Surg. 2020;28(1):46–51.
42. Martinez-Devesa P, Patiar S. Oral steroids for nasal polyps. Cochrane Database Syst Rev. 2011;7:CD005232.
43. Mainz JG, Koitschev A. Management of chronic rhinosinusitis in CF. J Cyst Fibros. 2009;8(Suppl 1):S10–4.
44. Cheng K, Ashby D, Smyth RL. Oral steroids for long-term use in cystic fibrosis. Cochrane Database Syst Rev. 2015;12:CD000407.
45. Nelson J, Karempelis P, Dunitz J, Hunter R, Boyer H. Pulmonary aspiration of sinus secretions in patients with cystic fibrosis. Int Forum Allergy Rhinol. 2018;8(3):385–8.
46. Aanaes K, von Buchwald C, Hjuler T, Skov M, Alanin M, Johansen HK. The effect of sinus surgery with intensive follow-up on pathogenic sinus bacteria in patients with cystic fibrosis. Am J Rhinol Allergy. 2013;27(1):e1–4.
47. Yamada T, Fujieda S, Mori S, Yamamoto H, Saito H. Macrolide treatment decreased the size of nasal polyps and IL-8 levels in nasal lavage. Am J Rhinol. 2000;14(3):143–8.
48. Majima Y. Clinical implications of the immunomodulatory effects of macrolides on sinusitis. Am J Med. 2004;117(Suppl 9A):20S–5S.

49. Gentzsch M, Mall MA. Ion channel modulators in cystic fibrosis. Chest. 2018;154(2):383–93.
50. Deeks ED. Lumacaftor/Ivacaftor: a review in cystic fibrosis. Drugs. 2016;76(12):1191–201.
51. Accurso FJ, Rowe SM, Clancy JP, Boyle MP, Dunitz JM, Durie PR, et al. Effect of VX-770 in persons with cystic fibrosis and the G551D-CFTR mutation. N Engl J Med. 2010;363(21):1991–2003.
52. Cho DY, Zhang S, Lazrak A, Grayson JW, Peña Garcia JA, Skinner DF, et al. Resveratrol and ivacaftor are additive G551D CFTR-channel potentiators: therapeutic implications for cystic fibrosis sinus disease. Int Forum Allergy Rhinol. 2019;9(1):100–5.
53. McCormick J, Cho DY, Lampkin B, Richman J, Hathorne H, Rowe SM, et al. Ivacaftor improves rhinologic, psychologic, and sleep-related quality of life in G551D cystic fibrosis patients. Int Forum Allergy Rhinol. 2019;9(3):292–7.
54. Sala MA, Jain M. Tezacaftor for the treatment of cystic fibrosis. Expert Rev Respir Med. 2018;12(9):725–32.
55. Middleton PG, Mall MA, Dřevínek P, Lands LC, McKone EF, Polineni D, et al. Elexacaftor-tezacaftor-ivacaftor for cystic fibrosis with a single Phe508del allele. N Engl J Med. 2019;381(19):1809–19.
56. Wainwright CE, Elborn JS, Ramsey BW. Lumacaftor-ivacaftor in patients with cystic fibrosis homozygous for Phe508del CFTR. N Engl J Med. 2015;373(18):1783–4.
57. Taylor-Cousar JL, Munck A, McKone EF, van der Ent CK, Moeller A, Simard C, et al. Tezacaftor-ivacaftor in patients with cystic fibrosis homozygous for Phe508del. N Engl J Med. 2017;377(21):2013–23.
58. Van Goor F, Hadida S, Grootenhuis PD, Burton B, Stack JH, Straley KS, et al. Correction of the F508del-CFTR protein processing defect in vitro by the investigational drug VX-809. Proc Natl Acad Sci U S A. 2011;108(46):18843–8.
59. Hoy SM. Elexacaftor/ivacaftor/tezacaftor: first approval. Drugs. 2019;79(18):2001–7.
60. Blount A, Zhang S, Chestnut M, Hixon B, Skinner D, Sorscher EJ, et al. Transepithelial ion transport is suppressed in hypoxic sinonasal epithelium. Laryngoscope. 2011;121(9):1929–34.
61. Mainz JG, Gerber A, Arnold C, Baumann J, Baumann I, Koitschev A. Rhinosinusitis in cystic fibrosis. HNO. 2015;63(11):809–20.
62. Banks C, Freeman L, Cho DY, Woodworth BA. Acquired cystic fibrosis transmembrane conductance regulator dysfunction. World J Otorhinolaryngol Head Neck Surg. 2018;4(3):193–9.
63. Cho DY, Woodworth BA. Acquired cystic fibrosis transmembrane conductance regulator deficiency. Adv Otorhinolaryngol. 2016;79:78–85.
64. Illing EA, Cho DY, Zhang S, Skinner DF, Dunlap QA, Sorscher EJ, et al. Chlorogenic acid activates CFTR-mediated Cl- secretion in mice and humans: therapeutic implications for chronic rhinosinusitis. Otolaryngol Head Neck Surg. 2015;153(2):291–7.
65. Woodworth BA. Resveratrol ameliorates abnormalities of fluid and electrolyte secretion in a hypoxia-induced model of acquired CFTR deficiency. Laryngoscope. 2015;125(Suppl 7):S1–S13.
66. Zhang S, Skinner D, Hicks SB, Bevensee MO, Sorscher EJ, Lazrak A, et al. Sinupret activates CFTR and TMEM16A-dependent transepithelial chloride transport and improves indicators of mucociliary clearance. PLoS One. 2014;9(8):e104090.
67. Zhang S, Smith N, Schuster D, Azbell C, Sorscher EJ, Rowe SM, et al. Quercetin increases cystic fibrosis transmembrane conductance regulator-mediated chloride transport and ciliary beat frequency: therapeutic implications for chronic rhinosinusitis. Am J Rhinol Allergy. 2011;25(5):307–12.
68. Azbell C, Zhang S, Skinner D, Fortenberry J, Sorscher EJ, Woodworth BA. Hesperidin stimulates cystic fibrosis transmembrane conductance regulator-mediated chloride secretion and ciliary beat frequency in sinonasal epithelium. Otolaryngol Head Neck Surg. 2010;143(3):397–404.
69. Virgin F, Zhang S, Schuster D, Azbell C, Fortenberry J, Sorscher EJ, et al. The bioflavonoid compound, sinupret, stimulates transepithelial chloride transport in vitro and in vivo. Laryngoscope. 2010;120(5):1051–6.

70. Alexander NS, Blount A, Zhang S, Skinner D, Hicks SB, Chestnut M, et al. Cystic fibrosis transmembrane conductance regulator modulation by the tobacco smoke toxin acrolein. Laryngoscope. 2012;122(6):1193–7.
71. Lambert JA, Raju SV, Tang LP, McNicholas CM, Li Y, Courville CA, et al. Cystic fibrosis transmembrane conductance regulator activation by roflumilast contributes to therapeutic benefit in chronic bronchitis. Am J Respir Cell Mol Biol. 2014;50(3):549–58.
72. Raju SV, Lin VY, Liu L, McNicholas CM, Karki S, Sloane PA, et al. The cystic fibrosis transmembrane conductance regulator potentiator ivacaftor augments mucociliary clearance abrogating cystic fibrosis transmembrane conductance regulator inhibition by cigarette smoke. Am J Respir Cell Mol Biol. 2017;56(1):99–108.
73. Sloane PA, Shastry S, Wilhelm A, Courville C, Tang LP, Backer K, et al. A pharmacologic approach to acquired cystic fibrosis transmembrane conductance regulator dysfunction in smoking related lung disease. PLoS One. 2012;7(6):e39809.
74. Robinson E, MacDonald KD, Slaughter K, McKinney M, Patel S, Sun C, et al. Lipid nanoparticle-delivered chemically modified mRNA restores chloride secretion in cystic fibrosis. Mol Ther. 2018;26(8):2034–46.
75. Johler SM, Rejman J, Guan S, Rosenecker J. Nebulisation of IVT mRNA complexes for intrapulmonary administration. PLoS One. 2015;10(9):e0137504.
76. Christopher Boyd A, Guo S, Huang L, Kerem B, Oren YS, Walker AJ, et al. New approaches to genetic therapies for cystic fibrosis. J Cyst Fibros. 2020;19(Suppl 1):S54–9.
77. Mention K, Santos L, Harrison PT. Gene and base editing as a therapeutic option for cystic fibrosis-learning from other diseases. Genes (Basel). 2019;10(5):387.
78. Cooney AL, McCray PB, Sinn PL. Cystic fibrosis gene therapy: looking back, looking forward. Genes (Basel). 2018;9(11):538.
79. Harvey R, Hannan SA, Badia L, Scadding G. Nasal saline irrigations for the symptoms of chronic rhinosinusitis. Cochrane Database Syst Rev. 2007;3:CD006394.
80. Elkins MR, Robinson M, Rose BR, Harbour C, Moriarty CP, Marks GB, et al. A controlled trial of long-term inhaled hypertonic saline in patients with cystic fibrosis. N Engl J Med. 2006;354(3):229–40.
81. Mainz JG, Schumacher U, Schädlich. K, Hentschel J, Koitschev C, Koitschev A, et al. Sino nasal inhalation of isotonic versus hypertonic saline (6.0%) in CF patients with chronic rhinosinusitis – results of a multicenter, prospective, randomized, double-blind, controlled trial. J Cyst Fibros. 2016;15(6):e57–66.
82. Safi C, Zheng Z, Dimango E, Keating C, Gudis DA. Chronic rhinosinusitis in cystic fibrosis: diagnosis and medical management. Med Sci (Basel). 2019;7(2):32.
83. Tran K, McCormack S. Intranasal corticosteroids for the management of chronic rhinosinusitis or nasal polyposis in cystic fibrosis: a review of clinical effectiveness. 2019.
84. Hadfield PJ, Rowe-Jones JM, Mackay IS. A prospective treatment trial of nasal polyps in adults with cystic fibrosis. Rhinology. 2000;38(2):63–5.
85. Bhalla RK, Payton K, Wright ED. Safety of budesonide in saline sinonasal irrigations in the management of chronic rhinosinusitis with polyposis: lack of significant adrenal suppression. J Otolaryngol Head Neck Surg. 2008;37(6):821–5.
86. Welch KC, Thaler ER, Doghramji LL, Palmer JN, Chiu AG. The effects of serum and urinary cortisol levels of topical intranasal irrigations with budesonide added to saline in patients with recurrent polyposis after endoscopic sinus surgery. Am J Rhinol Allergy. 2010;24(1):26–8.
87. Grayson JW, Harvey RJ. Topical corticosteroid irrigations in chronic rhinosinusitis. Int Forum Allergy Rhinol. 2019;9(S1):S9–S15.
88. Davidson TM, Murphy C, Mitchell M, Smith C, Light M. Management of chronic sinusitis in cystic fibrosis. Laryngoscope. 1995;105(4 Pt 1):354–8.
89. Shah GB, De Keyzer L, Russell JA, Halderman A. Treatment of chronic rhinosinusitis with dornase alfa in patients with cystic fibrosis: a systematic review. Int Forum Allergy Rhinol. 2018;8(6):729–36.

90. Han JK, Marple BF, Smith TL, Murr AH, Lanier BJ, Stambaugh JW, et al. Effect of steroid-releasing sinus implants on postoperative medical and surgical interventions: an efficacy meta-analysis. Int Forum Allergy Rhinol. 2012;2(4):271–9.

91. Han JK, Kern RC. Topical therapies for management of chronic rhinosinusitis: steroid implants. Int Forum Allergy Rhinol. 2019;9(S1):S22–S6.

92. Makadia HK, Siegel SJ. Poly Lactic-co-Glycolic Acid (PLGA) as biodegradable controlled drug delivery carrier. Polymers. 2011;3(3):1377–97.

93. Li PM, Downie D, Hwang PH. Controlled steroid delivery via bioabsorbable stent: safety and performance in a rabbit model. Am J Rhinol Allergy. 2009;23(6):591–6.

94. Cho DY, Hoffman K, Skinner D, Mackey C, Lim DJ, Alexander GC, et al. Tolerance and pharmacokinetics of a ciprofloxacin-coated sinus stent in a preclinical model. Int Forum Allergy Rhinol. 2017;7(4):352–8.

95. Cho DY, Lim DJ, Mackey C, Skinner D, Weeks C, Gill GS, et al. Preclinical therapeutic efficacy of the ciprofloxacin-eluting sinus stent for Pseudomonas aeruginosa sinusitis. Int Forum Allergy Rhinol. 2018;8(4):482–9.

96. Cho DY, Lim DJ, Mackey C, Weeks CG, Garcia JAP, Skinner D, et al. In-vitro evaluation of a ciprofloxacin- and ivacaftor-coated sinus stent against Pseudomonas aeruginosa biofilms. Int Forum Allergy Rhinol. 2019;9(5):486–92.

97. Cho DY, Lim DJ, Mackey C, Skinner D, Zhang S, McCormick J, et al. Ivacaftor, a cystic fibrosis transmembrane conductance regulator potentiator, enhances ciprofloxacin activity against Pseudomonas aeruginosa. Am J Rhinol Allergy. 2019;33(2):129–36.

98. Lim D-J, McCormick J, Skinner D, Zhang S, Elder JB, McLemore JG, et al. Controlled delivery of ciprofloxacin and ivacaftor via sinus stent in a preclinical model of Pseudomonas sinusitis. Int Forum Allergy Rhinol. 2019. https://doi.org/10.1002/alr.22514.

99. Zheng Z, Safi C, Gudis DA. Surgical management of chronic rhinosinusitis in cystic fibrosis. Med Sci (Basel). 2019;7(4):57.

100. Khalid AN, Mace J, Smith TL. Outcomes of sinus surgery in adults with cystic fibrosis. Otolaryngol Head Neck Surg. 2009;141(3):358–63.

101. Liang J, Higgins TS, Ishman SL, Boss EF, Benke JR, Lin SY. Surgical management of chronic rhinosinusitis in cystic fibrosis: a systematic review. Int Forum Allergy Rhinol. 2013;3(10):814–22.

102. Macdonald KI, Gipsman A, Magit A, Fandino M, Massoud E, Witterick IJ, et al. Endoscopic sinus surgery in patients with cystic fibrosis: a systematic review and meta-analysis of pulmonary function. Rhinology. 2012;50(4):360–9.

103. Aanaes K, Johansen HK, Skov M, Buchvald FF, Hjuler T, Pressler T, et al. Clinical effects of sinus surgery and adjuvant therapy in cystic fibrosis patients – can chronic lung infections be postponed? Rhinology. 2013;51(3):222–30.

104. Crockett DJ, Wilson KF, Meier JD. Perioperative strategies to improve sinus surgery outcomes in patients with cystic fibrosis: a systematic review. Otolaryngol Head Neck Surg. 2013;149(1):30–9.

105. Batra PS, Kern RC, Tripathi A, Conley DB, Ditto AM, Haines GK, et al. Outcome analysis of endoscopic sinus surgery in patients with nasal polyps and asthma. Laryngoscope. 2003;113(10):1703–6.

106. Virgin FW, Rowe SM, Wade MB, Gaggar A, Leon KJ, Young KR, et al. Extensive surgical and comprehensive postoperative medical management for cystic fibrosis chronic rhinosinusitis. Am J Rhinol Allergy. 2012;26(1):70–5.

107. Shatz A. Management of recurrent sinus disease in children with cystic fibrosis: a combined approach. Otolaryngol Head Neck Surg. 2006;135(2):248–52.

108. Khalfoun S, Tumin D, Ghossein M, Lind M, Hayes D, Kirkby S. Improved lung function after sinus surgery in cystic fibrosis patients with moderate obstruction. Otolaryngol Head Neck Surg. 2018;158(2):381–5.

109. Rosbe KW, Jones DT, Rahbar R, Lahiri T, Auerbach AD. Endoscopic sinus surgery in cystic fibrosis: do patients benefit from surgery? Int J Pediatr Otorhinolaryngol. 2001;61(2):113–9.

110. Triglia JM, Nicollas R. Nasal and sinus polyposis in children. Laryngoscope. 1997;107(7):963–6.
111. Kovell LC, Wang J, Ishman SL, Zeitlin PL, Boss EF. Cystic fibrosis and sinusitis in children: outcomes and socioeconomic status. Otolaryngol Head Neck Surg. 2011;145(1):146–53.
112. Jarrett WA, Militsakh O, Anstad M, Manaligod J. Endoscopic sinus surgery in cystic fibrosis: effects on pulmonary function and ideal body weight. Ear Nose Throat J. 2004;83(2):118–21.
113. Madonna D, Isaacson G, Rosenfeld RM, Panitch H. Effect of sinus surgery on pulmonary function in patients with cystic fibrosis. Laryngoscope. 1997;107(3):328–31.
114. Osborn AJ, Leung R, Ratjen F, James AL. Effect of endoscopic sinus surgery on pulmonary function and microbial pathogens in a pediatric population with cystic fibrosis. Arch Otolaryngol Head Neck Surg. 2011;137(6):542–7.
115. Luparello P, Lazio MS, Voltolini L, Borchi B, Taccetti G, Maggiore G. Outcomes of endoscopic sinus surgery in adult lung transplant patients with cystic fibrosis. Eur Arch Otorhinolaryngol. 2019;276(5):1341–7.
116. Leung MK, Rachakonda L, Weill D, Hwang PH. Effects of sinus surgery on lung transplantation outcomes in cystic fibrosis. Am J Rhinol. 2008;22(2):192–6.

Chapter 11
Bronchiectasis and Chronic Rhinosinusitis

Raymond Kim and Peter H. Hwang

> **Key Concepts**
> - Bronchiectasis is a term that describes a clinical end point of irreversible bronchial dilatation and destruction, rather than a distinct disease entity. The pathogenesis of bronchiectasis is heterogeneous, based on a diverse array of potential etiologies.
> - Chronic rhinosinusitis (CRS) and bronchiectasis share the hallmark feature of chronic airway inflammation and mucopurulence and have a significant epidemiological overlap.
> - Bronchiectasis patients with concurrent CRS have more frequent lower airway exacerbations than those without CRS. Surgical treatment of CRS improves sinonasal quality of life symptoms, but not pulmonary function.

Introduction

Definition/Description

Patients with chronic rhinosinusitis (CRS) can present with varying degrees of lower airway dysfunction. One of the more severe forms of lower airway disease that can present as a comorbid condition in CRS is bronchiectasis. The hallmark features of both CRS and bronchiectasis are chronic mucosal inflammation and excess mucus

R. Kim · P. H. Hwang (✉)
Division of Endoscopic Sinus & Skull Base Surgery, Department of Otolaryngology-Head & Neck Surgery, Stanford University School of Medicine, Stanford, CA, USA
e-mail: hwangph@stanford.edu

© Springer Nature Switzerland AG 2020
D. A. Gudis, R. J. Schlosser (eds.), *The Unified Airway*,
https://doi.org/10.1007/978-3-030-50330-7_11

production, differentiated anatomically by upper versus lower airway. Patients with bronchiectasis who have concurrent CRS have been shown to have significantly more lower airway exacerbations than those without CRS, even in the absence of upper airway flare. Patients with bronchiectasis and concurrent CRS also suffer significantly more detriment to quality of life [1, 2].

Bronchiectasis is defined by irreversible bronchial dilation and destruction, which manifests clinically as obstructive pulmonary disease marked by chronic cough and purulent sputum production. Bronchiectasis is a descriptive term for a clinical end point common to a variety of potential causes. It is a heterogeneous condition with multiple possible etiologies and associated comorbidities but also with a large proportion of idiopathic cases [3–5]. Thus, the term "bronchiectasis" is not defined by etiology. If there is sufficient clinical suspicion in a patient with persistent productive cough marked by purulent sputum, a high-resolution computer tomography (CT) imaging is performed to confirm the presence of bronchial dilatation, consistent with bronchiectasis [6]. While bronchiectasis is commonly observed in cystic fibrosis (CF), this chapter will focus on non-CF bronchiectasis.

Epidemiology

The incidence of non-CF bronchiectasis is 139 per 100,000 in the United States, with a higher incidence in women and a substantial increase in incidence with age (7/100,000 in subjects 18–35 years versus 812/100,000 in subjects ≥75 years) [7]. There has also been an observed increase in prevalence of 8.74% annually, although this is thought to be due to increasing awareness of the condition, as well as increased utilization of high-resolution CT imaging, rather than a true change in the pervasiveness of the disease [5]. Analysis of the largest US cohort of patients with bronchiectasis demonstrated that the most common demographic groups were non-Hispanic white women and lifelong nonsmokers [5].

In a study of patients with CRS, bronchiectasis was present in 16% of patients with CRS without nasal polyps (CRSsNP) without asthma, 5% of patients with CRS with nasal polyps (CRSwNP) without asthma, 24% of patients with CRSsNP and asthma, and 14% of patients with CRSwNP and asthma (versus 11% of asthmatics without CRS) [8]. Nearly half of bronchiectasis patients referred for nasal brush biopsy to rule out ciliary dyskinesia were found to have concurrent CRS [9]. Furthermore, a systematic review of patients with bronchiectasis identified a 62% prevalence of comorbid CRS, whose presence was associated with greater severity of bronchiectasis [1].

Etiology and Pathogenesis

In the last decade, the concept of the unified airway model has gained more evidence, where the entire upper and lower respiratory tract is considered an integrated system [10]. This model suggests that local inflammatory processes may generate systemic mediators stimulating all components of the unified airway and that exacerbations of disease in one portion of the airway could affect worsening of airway disease diffusely [10, 11].

In the upper airway, the defining feature of CRS is chronic inflammation of the sinonasal mucosa. This inflammation has been proposed to be secondary to inappropriate immune response to foreign antigens affecting the epithelial barrier [12]. However, the fundamental steps in the epithelial barrier disruption and the complex interactions with innate immunity are poorly understood. While a small proportion of patients may have systemic conditions such as primary ciliary dyskinesia, cystic fibrosis, or hypogammaglobulinemia, the majority are idiopathic.

The initial trigger that leads to the commencement of a chronic inflammatory state is unclear. Pathogens observed in the sinonasal cavities may be opportunistic manifestations of a defective epithelial barrier and local immune dysfunction, or they may be driving the inflammatory response. Increased T lymphocytes, eosinophils, basophils, neutrophils, and subepithelial collagen deposition have been observed in CRS [13]. Viruses, fungi, and bacteria have all been considered as potential instigators of upper airway epithelial barrier disruption. Viruses have been associated with both obstruction of the sinus ostiomeatal complex [9] and development of epithelial cell dysfunction [1]. Intranasal fungi have been postulated to exacerbate CRS through protease effects on nasal epithelial cells as well as activation of eosinophils and lymphocytes [10], but apart from allergic fungal rhinosinusitis, there is no clear evidence of fungal antigens targeting T or B cells in the sinonasal mucosa [10, 11]. Despite recent advances in our understanding of the bacterial microbiome in the sinuses, the pathogenic role of bacteria in CRS has yet to be elucidated. Bacterial biofilms [12] and subepithelial intramucosal bacteria may represent non-planktonic niches associated with sinus mucosa in CRS [13].

In the lower airway, the pathogenesis of bronchiectasis embodies a vicious cycle of chronic bronchial infection, inflammation, and impaired mucociliary clearance, which leads to permanent destruction and dilation of the bronchi and bronchioles [14]. Inflammatory infiltrates by lymphocytes and neutrophils, as well as increased presence of interleukins, are thought to be important contributors to bronchiectasis [15]. The functionality of neutrophils, for example, may be different in bronchiectasis patients, with unopposed elaboration of neutrophil elastases, greater production of myeloperoxidase, and greater neutrophil viability (reduced apoptosis) [16]. The sputum produced in bronchiectasis is notably more viscous, elastic, and hyperconcentrated compared to normal controls, owing to greater production of mucins and sputum solids. Bacterial pathogens also contribute to the purulent milieu, notably *Pseudomonas aeruginosa, Haemophilus influenza, Staphylococcus aureus*, nontuberculous mycobacteria, and fungi [17]. In discussing the pathogenesis, however, one needs to consider the fact that bronchiectasis is not a physiologic condition per se, but rather a clinical end point resulting from a varied array of potential etiologies. The possible etiologies of bronchiectasis include idiopathic, chronic airway obstruction from foreign body or tumor; a complication of previous lower airway bacterial or mycobacterial infections; deficits in host defenses, such as common variable immunodeficiency, or rheumatic disease; or overlapping conditions such as cystic fibrosis, severe chronic obstructive pulmonary disease (COPD), primary ciliary dyskinesia (PCD), asthma, or allergic bronchopulmonary aspergillosis (ABPA) [2, 4, 18]. While each of these respiratory conditions has its own pathogenesis, the diagnosis of bronchiectasis does not predicate the disease mechanism. Furthermore, the thin-slice CT scans, by which bronchiectasis is diagnosed, neither are specific or sensitive nor have any influence on determining the prognosis or treatment recommendations [17].

In discussing the pathogenesis from a unified airway perspective, the overlapping prevalence of CRS in patients with bronchiectasis secondary to CF or PCD is essentially universal [19]. However, whereas CF and PCD have defined epithelial abnormalities that affect both the upper and lower airways, in patients with bronchiectasis without CF or PCD, the pathogenetic link to CRS is varied and often unclear [2]. Certain conditions such as immunodeficiency and autoimmune disease may independently affect the paranasal sinuses and bronchi/bronchioles. In such cases, the presence of concurrent sinusitis and bronchiectasis may not represent a causative relationship but rather a comorbid relationship. For other etiologies, the determinants of relatedness between sinonasal disease and bronchiectasis are not well-defined. For example, although neutrophil infiltration has been described in classic bronchiectasis [12], peripheral eosinophil and IgE levels have been shown to be higher in bronchiectasis patients with CRS compared to bronchiectasis patients without CRS [20]. Conditions that have been postulated to contribute to both sinonasal disease and bronchiectasis include atopy, vitamin D deficiency, and heterozygosity for the cystic fibrosis transmembrane regulator (CFTR) gene [21–23].

Clinical Presentation

Patient Demographic and Medical Context

In a large retrospective cohort study of 900 patients with bronchiectasis, 45% were found to have concurrent CRS, and in this population, significant associations with allergic rhinitis, antibody deficiency, asthma, and gastroesophageal reflux disease (GERD) were identified when compared to those without CRS [24]. A majority of bronchiectasis patients with or without CRS were female, consistent with findings of the US Bronchiectasis Research Registry [5].

Signs and Symptoms

There are no pathognomonic signs or symptoms associated with concurrent CRS and bronchiectasis. Independent familiarity with the symptom profiles for CRS and for bronchiectasis is therefore necessary in order to make the correct diagnoses. For physicians more familiar with diagnosing CRS, the presence of a persistent productive cough, purulent sputum, and chronic dyspnea should raise concern for possible bronchiectasis.

Diagnostics

Typical Physical Examination Findings

Upper and lower airway examination findings of patients with concurrent non-CF bronchiectasis and chronic rhinosinusitis do not appear to deviate from those found in the respective conditions in isolation. There has not been a specific phenotypic CRS subtype that has been associated with bronchiectasis, although one group reported higher prevalence of nasal polyps in idiopathic and postinfectious bronchiectasis patients with CRS [25].

Typical Radiographic Features

The British Society guidelines for radiologic evaluation of bronchiectasis recommend a baseline chest x-ray for clinical suspicion of bronchiectasis and a thin-slice CT to diagnose the condition as per the following criteria [6]:

- One or more of the following:

  - Bronchoarterial ratio >1 (internal airway lumen versus adjacent pulmonary artery)
  - Lack of tapering
  - Airway visibility within 1 cm of costal pleural surface or touching mediastinal pleura

- With following indirect signs commonly associated with bronchiectasis:

  - Bronchial wall thickening
  - Mucus impaction
  - Mosaic perfusion/air trapping on expiratory CT

For CRS, CT scan remains the gold standard for radiologic diagnosis [26]. The presence of mucosal thickening, obstructed sinus outlet pathways, and/or presence of polyps may be seen in CRS both with and without bronchiectasis. There are no distinguishing CT findings unique to CRS with bronchiectasis, but CT severity score may be higher in those patients with concurrent bronchiectasis [27–30].

Medical Management and Outcomes with Overview of Evidence

Given the broad range of therapeutic options for bronchiectasis as well as for CRS, this discussion will be limited to therapies that may be common to treatment of both entities.

Systemic Medical Therapy

(i) *Bronchiectasis* [4, 6, 31]

- *Oral antibiotics:* Oral antibiotics can serve as an alternative to inhaled antibiotics when topical therapies are not tolerated. Macrolides, despite a more limited antibacterial spectrum, may be beneficial for their anti-inflammatory effects (Th-1, neutrophilic), as well as for their potential mucolytic and anti-biofilm effects. For an acute exacerbation of bronchiectasis, a 14-day course has been recommended by a historic guideline [32], and there is no clear evidence for shorter or longer course duration. For patients with more than three exacerbations per year, long-term (≥3 months) antibiotics are recommended; macrolides (azithromycin or erythromycin) and doxycycline, where macrolides are not tolerated, have all demonstrated efficacy in reducing exacerbation frequency. However, the randomized trials that have examined these therapies have varied in duration (3–12 months) and dose of the antibiotics (250 mg azithromycin daily, 500 mg or 250 mg three times per week, or erythromycin 400 mg twice daily).
- *Intravenous antibiotics:* Intravenous antibiotics may be used for acute exacerbations. Also, a significant reduction in exacerbation frequency has been shown in patients with severe bronchiectasis of more than five exacerbations a year, where cyclical culture-directed antibiotics (e.g. ceftazidime, tazobactam/piperacillin, aztreonam) were used for 14 days per course, 8 weekly. There is also low-level evidence to suggest that IV antibiotics followed by inhaled antibiotics may lead to *P. aeruginosa* eradication with resulting clinical improvement, although with unchanged lung functions.
- *Oral corticosteroids:* There have been no randomized controlled trials for the use of oral corticosteroids in the management of acute exacerbations of

bronchiectasis or for management of baseline symptoms. However, they may be used in patients with other conditions, such as chronic asthma, inflammatory bowel disease, and COPD.

- *Vaccination:* Despite limited studies examining the benefit of vaccines, annual influenza and polysaccharide pneumococcal vaccination are recommended based on a favorable risk-benefit ratio.

(ii) *CRS* [33, 34]

- *Oral antibiotics:* Similar to treatment for bronchiectasis, long-term macrolide antibiotics have been shown through Level 1 evidence to benefit patients with CRS, leading to significant symptom and endoscopic score improvement. However, the benefit was equivalent to intranasal topical corticosteroid use and the benefit not maintained after cessation. There is no evidence-based recommendation for longer-term non-macrolide antibiotics.
- *Oral corticosteroids:* In CRSwNP patients, several double-blinded placebo-controlled randomized controlled studies have demonstrated at least short-term symptom improvements, including improvement in olfaction and visible reduction in polyp volume. Duration of effect may last for several months when used in conjunction with topical corticosteroids. Despite common use in CRSsNP patients, there is limited evidence to support this practice. The systemic absorption and associated adverse effects preclude prolonged systemic corticosteroid treatment.

Topical Medical Therapy

(i) *Bronchiectasis* [4, 6, 31]

- *Corticosteroids:* While large randomized controlled trials are lacking, inhaled corticosteroids have not demonstrated clinically significant benefit in cough-related quality of life or lung function and are not recommended for bronchiectasis. However, topical corticosteroid use may be indicated in patients with comorbid asthma or COPD.
- *Antibiotics:* Moderate-quality evidence supports the use of long-term topical antibiotics (e.g., inhaled colistin or gentamicin) for patients colonized with *Pseudomonas aeruginosa*, if having three or more exacerbations per year. There is also limited evidence to support long-term topical antibiotics for prophylaxis in those without *Pseudomonas aeruginosa*, where oral antibiotic prophylaxis is unable to be used.
- *Mucoactive treatments:* Mucoactive medications directly impact the clearance of mucus from airways, and their classes of action include expectorants, mucolytics, mucokinetics, and mucoregulators. Recombinant human DNase, a mucolytic, has demonstrated an increase in exacerbation frequency, while nebulizing with iso- or hypertonic saline improved cough-related quality of

life indices. Mucoactive treatment trial may be considered in patients with sputum expectoration difficulty.

(ii) *CRS* [33, 34]

- *Corticosteroids:* There is high-level and quality evidence of long-term efficacy and safety for topical corticosteroid sprays, and it is the mainstay medical treatment for CRS. Off-label use of corticosteroid irrigations has gained popularity, with several studies supporting a beneficial effect. Steroid-eluting bioabsorbable implants are relatively new method of delivery, and efficacy has been demonstrated, including significant improvement in olfaction. They have also been shown to be well-tolerated with no increased locoregional or systemic adverse outcomes.
- *Antibiotics:* Although high-volume saline rinsing with mupirocin added demonstrates superior ability to eradicate *S. aureus* compared to oral amoxicillin/clavulanate, placebo-controlled randomized controlled studies demonstrate clinically nonrelevant improvement in symptoms and endoscopic scores.
- *Mucoactive treatments:* Isotonic saline irrigation in CRS patients has been demonstrated to be beneficial in large-scale Level 1 studies. However, there is limited evidence to demonstrate large volume being more effective than delivery via sprays. Hypertonic saline rinses and additives such as xylitol and manuka honey may have some benefit but require larger-scale studies to validate their use. Surfactants have a limited role given reports of nasal irritation and hyposmia in clinical trials.

Emerging Therapies

In both bronchiectasis and CRS, there are increasing insights into the underlying immune processes leading to the hallmark feature of chronic inflammation. Classifying these conditions according to inflammatory endotype rather than by traditional phenotypical presentations has opened doors to targeted immunomodulatory and disease-modifying agents, tailored to the individual patient.

Given the dominance of neutrophilic inflammation in bronchiectasis, emerging tailored therapies include targeting neutrophils (e.g., neutrophil elastase) [35] or the more upstream bone marrow-targeted inhibition (e.g., dipeptidyl peptidase 1 inhibitor) [31] or use of various immunomodulatory drugs such as vitamin D and granulocyte-macrophage colony-stimulating factors [36]. Beyond endotyping, "treatable traits" is a term to describe characterizing individual patients according to their genetic, biomarker, phenotypic, or psychosocial characteristics [17]. These efforts recognize the heterogeneity of the various airway diseases and aim to offer personalized therapeutic options for patients [2, 4, 17, 18].

Similarly in CRS, endotyping patients by inflammatory profile (e.g., IgE, eosinophils, IL-4, IL-5, IL-13) is opening doors to novel therapeutic options [34, 37, 38]. For example, the biologic agent dupilumab (anti-IL-4 and anti-IL-13) was recently approved by the US Food and Drug Administration and the European Medicines Agency for treatment of chronic rhinosinusitis with polyposis.

Surgical Management and Outcomes with Overview of Evidence

(i) *Bronchiectasis* [19]

Surgery for bronchiectasis consists of partial lung resection or transplantation. Partial resection is reserved for patients presenting with severe localized disease or frequent exacerbations despite medical optimization of all other aspects of care. Other indications include uncontrolled hemorrhage or destructed lung partially obstructed by a tumor or foreign body. In a case series of 790 bronchiectasis patients undergoing partial lung resection, 75% experienced clinical improvement or resolution of symptoms over a 4-year follow-up period.

Patients could be considered for lung transplant if under 65 years of age with <30% FEV1 or rapid deterioration or additional features such as severe hemoptysis, pulmonary hypertension, or intensive care unit admissions. In a select group of patients with tracheobronchomegaly, a stabilizing procedure with a tracheobronchoplasty or stent placement may improve mucus clearance and therefore lung function [39].

(ii) *CRS* [2]

There are relatively few studies examining the outcomes of endoscopic sinus surgery in patients with chronic rhinosinusitis and bronchiectasis. A retrospective review of patients undergoing endoscopic surgery for CRS who had a concurrent diagnosis of bronchiectasis revealed significant reduction in the Sinonasal Outcome Test-22 (SNOT-22) symptom score, with durable improvement over 3 years [40]. Despite symptomatic improvement, there was no observed improvement in their pulmonary function tests.

Another review compared surgical with medical therapy of CRS in patients with comorbid bronchiectasis over a 6-month follow-up period [41]. Although both cohorts showed improvements in sinus symptom scores and sinus CT scores, the cohort undergoing sinus surgery had a greater degree of symptomatic and radiologic improvement in sinus disease. From a pulmonary standpoint, the surgical cohort showed a significantly greater reduction in pulmonary exacerbations versus the medical cohort; however, neither group showed improvements in pulmonary function testing.

Impact of Rhinologic Interventions on Bronchiectasis

Under the unified airway hypothesis, there is some evidence that surgical optimization of the upper airway can benefit lower airway function. In patients with asthma, sinus surgery has been associated with significant improvement in quality of life [42] and pulmonary function [24]. In patients with CF, endoscopic sinus surgery has been associated with significant quality of life improvement [5], as well as a reduction in respiratory tract infections and antibiotic requirements in lung transplant patients with CF [25].

However, in CRS patients with non-CF bronchiectasis, the pulmonary response to sinus surgery appears to be disappointingly limited. As described in the previous section, although the frequency of pulmonary exacerbations may improve, sinus surgery has not shown to improve pulmonary function. The lack of improvement in objective pulmonary function testing is consistent with the irreversibility of the destructive airway dilatation seen in bronchiectasis, which is at odds with the potential reversibility of the inflammatory changes seen in chronic rhinosinusitis. Patients with non-CF bronchiectasis undergoing sinus surgery should be counselled accordingly to establish realistic expectations for clinical prognosis.

Case Presentation

A 35-year-old female elementary school teacher was referred for management of chronic rhinosinusitis. She had daily nasal congestion, thick rhinorrhea, and facial pressure. Her past medical history was notable for frequent hospitalizations for pneumonia as a child, as well as recurrent otitis media requiring several myringotomies with tympanostomy tube placement. At the age of 16, the patient was evaluated for chronic productive cough and dyspnea and underwent a chest CT scan. The CT scan was notable for dextrocardia and bronchiectasis (Fig. 11.1).

She subsequently underwent ciliary biopsy of the nasal mucosa, which revealed abnormal ciliary ultrastructure with absent dynein arms on transmission electron microscopy. The patient was diagnosed with primary ciliary dyskinesia, having the classic triad of bronchiectasis, situs inversus, and sinusitis (Kartagener syndrome).

After being diagnosed with PCD as a teenager, she managed her sinonasal symptoms conservatively with saline irrigations and occasional antibiotics and nasal steroid sprays. However, her symptoms gradually became more severe through her early adulthood years, and a CT scan of the sinuses was then obtained, showing pansinusitis (Fig. 11.2).

After completion of a trial of appropriate medical therapy without improvement, the patient underwent endoscopic sinus surgery of all sinuses, including maxillary sinus mega-antrostomies, which were created to facilitate gravity-dependent drainage of the maxillary sinuses. Her preoperative pulmonary function test showed an FEV1 of 1.5L (61%) and FVC of 2.69L (84%).

Fig. 11.1 High-resolution CT thorax. High-resolution CT demonstrates situs inversus with dextrocardia (★), marked bronchiectasis and cicatricial atelectasis with consolidation of the right lower lobe, and scattered areas of bronchiectasis in the left lung (▲)

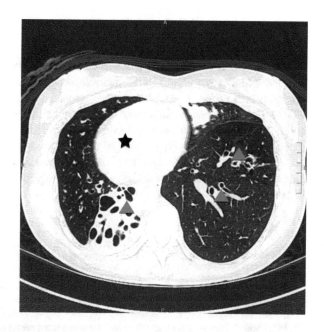

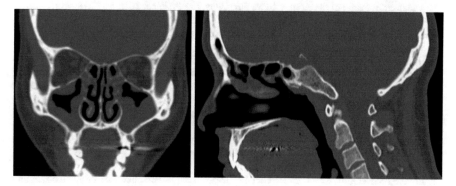

Fig. 11.2 CT paranasal sinuses. Pansinusitis with hyperostosis around the sphenoid sinus, indicating chronicity of the inflammation

The patient tolerated general anesthesia well, having been medically optimized by the pulmonology service preoperatively, and she was discharged to home on the day of surgery. Her postoperative course was notable for significant improvement in her sinonasal symptoms, with reduction of her SNOT-22 score from 39/110 preoperatively to 13/110 at her 6-month postoperative visit. Her postoperative pulmonary function tests were not improved, but were stable. She continues to do well from a sinonasal and pulmonary standpoint at 1 year postoperatively.

Conclusion

Bronchiectasis is an irreversibly destructive distal airway disease with heterogeneous etiologies of chronic inflammation. Multiple conditions can predispose to bronchiectasis, such as asthma, cystic fibrosis, primary ciliary dyskinesia, and COPD, but there also exists a large proportion of idiopathic cases. Although CRS and bronchiectasis are often diagnosed as comorbid conditions, there is not a clear link of causality despite the concept of unified airway disease. Although sinus surgery can improve sinonasal quality of life, the irreversible structural damage associated with bronchiectasis limits the potential beneficial impact of sinus surgery on lung function.

References

1. Handley E, Nicolson CH, Hew M, Lee AL. Prevalence and clinical implications of chronic rhinosinusitis in people with bronchiectasis: a systematic review. J Allergy Clin Immunol Pract. 2019;7(6):2004–2012.e1. https://doi.org/10.1016/j.jaip.2019.02.026.
2. Polverino E, Dimakou K, Hurst J, et al. The overlap between bronchiectasis and chronic airway diseases: state of the art and future directions. Eur Respir J. 2018;52(3):1800328. https://doi.org/10.1183/13993003.00328-2018.
3. King P, Holdsworth S, Freezer N, Holmes P. Bronchiectasis. Intern Med J. 2006;36(11):729–37. https://doi.org/10.1111/j.1445-5994.2006.01219.x.
4. Hacken ten N, Kerstjens H, Postma D. Bronchiectasis. BMJ Clin Evid. 2008;1(1507).
5. Aksamit TR, O'Donnell AE, Barker A, et al. Adult patients with bronchiectasis: a first look at the US Bronchiectasis Research Registry. Chest. 2017;151(5):982–92. https://doi.org/10.1016/j.chest.2016.10.055.
6. Hill AT, Sullivan AL, Chalmers JD, et al. British Thoracic Society Guideline for bronchiectasis in adults. Thorax. 2019;74(Suppl 1):1–69. https://doi.org/10.1136/thoraxjnl-2018-212463.
7. Weycker D, Hansen GL, Seifer FD. Prevalence and incidence of noncystic fibrosis bronchiectasis among US adults in 2013. Chron Respir Dis. 2017;14(4):377–84. https://doi.org/10.1177/1479972317709649.
8. Bose S, Stevens W, Li N, et al. Unified airway theory: association of bronchiectasis and chronic rhinosinusitis. J Allergy Clin Immunol. 2016;137(Supplement):AB284. https://doi.org/10.1016/j.jaci.2015.12.1176.
9. McCormick JP, Weeks CG, Rivers NJ, et al. Prevalence of chronic rhinosinusitis in bronchiectasis patients suspected of ciliary dyskinesia. Int Forum Allergy Rhinol. 2019;9(12):1430–5. https://doi.org/10.1002/alr.22414.
10. Krouse JH. The unified airway--conceptual framework. Otolaryngol Clin North Am. 2008;41(2):257–66–v. https://doi.org/10.1016/j.otc.2007.11.002.
11. Passalacqua G. United airways disease: therapeutic aspects. Thorax. 2000;55(90002):26S–27. https://doi.org/10.1136/thorax.55.suppl_2.S26.
12. Kern RC, Conley DB, Walsh W, et al. Perspectives on the etiology of chronic rhinosinusitis: an immune barrier hypothesis. Am J Rhinol. 2012;22(6):549–59. https://doi.org/10.2500/ajr.2008.22.3228.
13. Sobol SE, Sobol SE, Fukakusa M, et al. Inflammation and remodeling of the sinus mucosa in children and adults with chronic sinusitis. Laryngoscope. 2003;113(3):410–4. https://doi.org/10.1097/00005537-200303000-00004.

14. Ha KR, Psaltis AJ, Tan L, Wormald P-J. A sheep model for the study of biofilms in rhinosinus-itis. Am J Rhinol. 2007;21(3):339–45.
15. Tieu DD, Kern RC, Schleimer RP. Alterations in epithelial barrier function and host defense responses in chronic rhinosinusitis. J Allergy Clin Immunol. 2009;124(1):37–42. https://doi.org/10.1016/j.jaci.2009.04.045.
16. Ramsey KA, Chen ACH, Radicioni G, et al. Airway mucus hyperconcentration in non-cystic fibrosis bronchiectasis. Am J Respir Crit Care Med. 2020;201(6):661–70. https://doi.org/10.1164/rccm.201906-1219OC.
17. Society ER. "Is bronchiectasis really a disease?" Michal Shteinberg, Patrick A. Flume and James D. Chalmers. Eur Respir Rev 2020; 29: 190051. Eur Respir Rev. 2020;29(155):195051. https://doi.org/10.1183/16000617.5051-2019.
18. Chalmers JD, Chotirmall SH. Bronchiectasis: new therapies and new perspectives. Lancet Respir Med. 2018;6(9):715–26. https://doi.org/10.1016/S2213-2600(18)30053-5.
19. Yii ACA, Tay T-R, Choo XN, Koh MSY, Tee AKH, Wang D-Y. Precision medicine in united airways disease: a "treatable traits" approach. Allergy. 2018;73(10):1964–78. https://doi.org/10.1111/all.13496.
20. Ebbens FA, Fokkens WJ. The mold conundrum in chronic rhinosinusitis: where do we stand today? Curr Allergy Asthma Rep. 2008;8(2):93–101.
21. Mac Aogáin M, Tiew PY, Lim AYH, et al. Distinct "immunoallertypes" of disease and high frequencies of sensitization in non-cystic fibrosis bronchiectasis. Am J Respir Crit Care Med. 2019;199(7):842–53. https://doi.org/10.1164/rccm.201807-1355OC.
22. Bienvenu T, Sermet-Gaudelus I, Burgel P-R, et al. Cystic fibrosis transmembrane conductance regulator channel dysfunction in non-cystic fibrosis bronchiectasis. Am J Respir Crit Care Med. 2010;181(10):1078–84. https://doi.org/10.1164/rccm.200909-1434OC.
23. Chalmers JD, McHugh BJ, Docherty C, Govan JRW, Hill AT. Vitamin-D deficiency is asso-ciated with chronic bacterial colonisation and disease severity in bronchiectasis. Thorax. 2013;68(1):39–47. https://doi.org/10.1136/thoraxjnl-2012-202125.
24. Somani SN, Kwah JH, Yeh C, et al. Prevalence and characterization of chronic rhinosinusitis in patients with non-cystic fibrosis bronchiectasis at a tertiary care center in the United States. Int Forum Allergy Rhinol. 2019;9(12):1424–9. https://doi.org/10.1002/alr.22436.
25. Guilemany JM, Angrill J, Alobid I, et al. United airways again: high prevalence of rhi-nosinusitis and nasal polyps in bronchiectasis. Allergy. 2009;64(5):790–7. https://doi.org/10.1111/j.1398-9995.2008.01892.x.
26. Psaltis AJ, Ha KR, Beule AG, Tan LW, Tan LW, Wormald P-J. Confocal scanning laser microscopy evidence of biofilms in patients with chronic rhinosinusitis. Laryngoscope. 2007;117(7):1302–6. https://doi.org/10.1097/MLG.0b013e31806009b0.
27. Clement S, Vaudaux P, Francois P, et al. Evidence of an intracellular reservoir in the nasal mucosa of patients with recurrent Staphylococcus aureus rhinosinusitis. J Infect Dis. 2005;192:1023–8.
28. Niederfuhr A, Kirsche H, Deutschle T, Poppert S, Riechelmann H, Wellinghausen N. Staphylococcus aureus in nasal lavage and biopsy of patients with chronic rhinosinusitis. Allergy. 2008;63(10):1359–67. https://doi.org/10.1111/j.1398-9995.2008.01798.x.
29. Corriveau M-N, Zhang N, Holtappels G, Van Roy N, Bachert C. Detection of Staphylococcus aureus in nasal tissue with peptide nucleic acid-fluorescence in situ hybridization. Am J Rhinol Allergy. 2009;23(5):461–5. https://doi.org/10.2500/ajra.2009.23.3367.
30. Wood AJ, Fraser JD, Swift S, Patterson-Emanuelson EAC, Amirapu S, Douglas RG. Intramucosal bacterial microcolonies exist in chronic rhinosinusitis without inducing a local immune response. Am J Rhinol Allergy. 2012;26(4):265–70. https://doi.org/10.2500/ajra.2012.26.3779.
31. Polverino E, Goeminne PC, McDonnell MJ, et al. European Respiratory Society guidelines for the management of adult bronchiectasis. Eur Respir J. 2017;50(3):1700629. https://doi.org/10.1183/13993003.00629-2017.

32. Pasteur MC, Bilton D, Hill AT, British Thoracic Society Non-CF Bronchiectasis Guideline Group. British Thoracic Society guideline for non-CF bronchiectasis. Thorax. 2010;65(7):577. https://doi.org/10.1136/thx.2010.142778.
33. Orlandi RR, Kingdom TT, Hwang PH, et al. International consensus statement on allergy and rhinology: rhinosinusitis. Int Forum Allergy Rhinol. 2016;6 Suppl 1(S1):S22–S209. https://doi.org/10.1002/alr.21695.
34. Fokkens WJ, Lund VJ, Hopkins C, et al. European position paper on rhinosinusitis and nasal polyps 2020. Rhinology. 2020;58(Suppl S29):1–464. https://doi.org/10.4193/Rhin20.600.
35. Gramegna A, Amati F, Terranova L, et al. Neutrophil elastase in bronchiectasis. Respir Res. 2017;18(1):211–3. https://doi.org/10.1186/s12931-017-0691-x.
36. Gaga M, Bentley AM, Humbert M, et al. Increases in CD4+ T lymphocytes, macrophages, neutrophils and interleukin 8 positive cells in the airways of patients with bronchiectasis. Thorax. 1998;53(8):685–91. https://doi.org/10.1136/thx.53.8.685.
37. Husain Q, Sedaghat AR. Understanding and clinical relevance of chronic rhinosinusitis endotypes. Clin Otolaryngol. 2019;44(6):887–97. https://doi.org/10.1111/coa.13455.
38. Wang C, Zhang L. Use of biologics in chronic sinusitis with nasal polyps. Curr Opin Allergy Clin Immunol. 2019;19(4):365–72. https://doi.org/10.1097/ACI.0000000000000540.
39. Odell DD, Shah A, Gangadharan SP, et al. Airway stenting and tracheobronchoplasty improve respiratory symptoms in Mounier-Kuhn syndrome. Chest. 2011;140(4):867–73. https://doi.org/10.1378/chest.10-2010.
40. Kanjanaumporn J, Hwang PH. Effect of endoscopic sinus surgery on bronchiectasis patients with chronic rhinosinusitis. Am J Rhinol Allergy. 2018;32(5):432–9. https://doi.org/10.1177/1945892418793539.
41. Wang Y, Yang H-B. Effects of functional endoscopic sinus surgery on the treatment of bronchiectasis combined with chronic rhino-sinusitis. Acta Otolaryngol. 2016;136(8):860–3. https://doi.org/10.3109/00016489.2016.1157730.
42. Shteinberg M, Nassrallah N, Jrbashyan J, Uri N, Stein N, Adir Y. Upper airway involvement in bronchiectasis is marked by early onset and allergic features. ERJ Open Res. 2018;4(1):00115–2017. https://doi.org/10.1183/23120541.00115-2017.

Chapter 12
Primary Ciliary Dyskinesia

Mikkel Christian Alanin

Key Concepts
- CRS is a hallmark of primary ciliary dyskinesia (PCD).
- There is limited evidence to support isolated medical management for PCD CRS at this time.
- Endoscopic sinus surgery (ESS) in combination with medical therapy can improve both sinonasal and pulmonary outcome measures.

Definition

The first case of primary ciliary dyskinesia (PCD) was published in the medical literature in 1904 [1]. In 1933, Kartagener published a case series of four patients with situs inversus, bronchiectasis, and chronic rhinosinusitis [2], and this clinical triad was then termed "Kartagener's syndrome," which is still encountered in the medical nomenclature today.

In 1976, the first studies using electron microscopy (EM) in patients with PCD demonstrated that the respiratory cilia were immotile due to structural defects [3]. Consequently, the disease was renamed as "immotile cilia syndrome." Subsequent studies have demonstrated that in some patients with PCD the cilia are not immotile but rather have ineffective cilia beat patterns. Therefore, the disorder is now termed "primary ciliary dyskinesia" (PCD) [4]. PCD is in distinction from secondary ciliary dyskinesia, which is ciliary dysfunction secondary to airway infection, inflammation, or mucostasis, or other forms of impaired mucociliary clearance.

M. C. Alanin (✉)
Department of Otorhinolaryngology, Rigshospitalet, Copenhagen, Denmark

© Springer Nature Switzerland AG 2020
D. A. Gudis, R. J. Schlosser (eds.), *The Unified Airway*,
https://doi.org/10.1007/978-3-030-50330-7_12

Epidemiology

The tentative prevalence of PCD is 1:15,000. Mild phenotypes of PCD may remain undiagnosed, and the true prevalence may therefore be higher [5]. PCD is primarily inherited in an autosomal recessive pattern, and genetic mutations in more than 30 genes responsible for the structure or function of cilia have been identified as pathogenetic. In ethnic groups with high rates of consanguinity, such as the Amish communities in the United States, the incidence is higher [6]. Genetic testing can currently identify approximately two-thirds of all patients with PCD [7].

Pathogenesis

PCD is inherited in an autosomal recessive pattern. Over 30 PCD-causing genetic mutations have been identified. Ciliated pseudostratified columnar epithelium in the respiratory tract, together with the mucus layer, is the dominant factors responsible for mucociliary clearance. An example of abnormal ciliary ultrastructure is shown in Fig. 12.1.

Clinical Presentation

PCD is primarily an oto-sino-pulmonary disease. In infancy, PCD may present with neonatal respiratory distress [8]. In children and adolescents, conductive hearing loss due to otitis media with effusion (OME) [9] is very common, and it can persist into adulthood. Additional chronic symptoms include cough, recurrent acute rhinosinusitis, and chronic rhinosinusitis (CRS) [10]. Acute and chronic lung infections can lead to structural lung parenchymal damage resulting in bronchiectasis, gradually declining lung function, and in severely affected patients end-stage lung disease requiring lung transplantation or ultimately death [11]. The median age of death has been reported to be 65 years [12]. Almost half of patients with PCD have situs inversus as well, and congenital heart defects are observed in 5% of PCD patients [13]. Subfertility or infertility is common due to effects of cilia dysfunction in the fallopian tubes and structural defects in the tail of the sperm cell.

Diagnosis of PCD is a clinical challenge. Nasal nitric oxide is extremely low in the vast majority of patients with PCD and is useful as a screening test [14]. A definitive diagnosis is based on the presence of a characteristic clinical phenotype combined with disease-specific EM changes (Fig. 12.1), characteristic ciliary movement abnormalities on high-speed video microscopy, or a verified PCD genetic defect [14].

On ENT examination, it is common to find otitis media with effusion (OME). Studies report that more than 80% of PCD patients have OME, which can persist into adulthood [9]. Many practitioners have refrained from inserting ventilation tubes in patients with PCD with persistent OME as it can lead to ongoing otorrhea. However, newer studies have questioned the basis for this recommendation [15], and no prospective studies have assessed this management or evaluated the impact

Fig. 12.1 (**a**) Drawing of a respiratory motile cilium – simplified. Normal motile cilia contain nine outer doublets of microtubules ★ and a central pair ♛. This is called the 9+2 axonemal structure. From the doublet microtubules, inner ✿ and outer ✹ dynein arms originate. The doublets are connected with nexin links ♤, and the doublet connects to the central pair via radial spokes ◇. (**b**) Electron microscopy of a patient with a transposition defect as one example leading to primary ciliary dyskinesia. There is no central pair, only doublets, and one of them is transpositioned to a central position

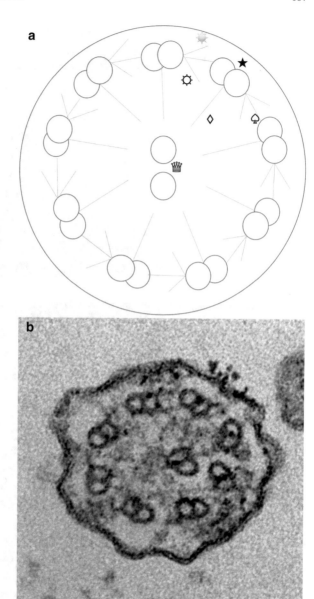

of topical steroid ear drops in PCD. Nevertheless, until this has been investigated further, conservative management of OME with hearing aids is a reasonable treatment option. If this option fails, ventilation tubes may be indicated.

CRS is a hallmark of PCD, and many studies have found a prevalence exceeding 70% [10, 16]. Nasal polyps can be found in 15–56% of adult PCD patients (Fig. 12.2) [10, 17] and can appear in children as well [18]. If polyps are visualized in any child, PCD or cystic fibrosis (CF) should be among the differential diagnoses. Thick and stagnant white mucus, due to impaired mucociliary clearance, is a common finding on nasal endoscopy (Fig. 12.2). As in patients with CF, the sinuses in PCD

Fig. 12.2 Nasal polyps
and characteristic sticky
white secretions in patient
with PCD

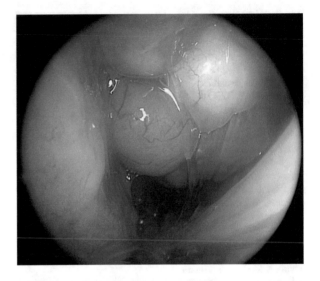

Fig. 12.3 Abnormal sinus
anatomy. Hypoplastic
right frontal sinus. Aplastic
left frontal sinus in adult
patient with PCD

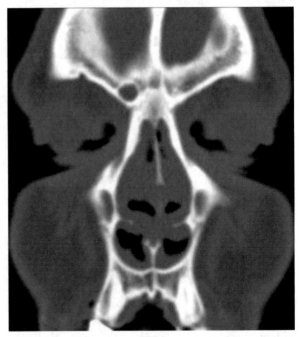

patients may function as a bacterial reservoir for Gram-negative bacteria including *Pseudomonas aeruginosa*. From the sinuses, the bacteria can migrate to a colonize the lungs repeatedly [19, 20].

CT opacities on sinus scans are ubiquitous in adult patients with PCD [20]. Abnormal sinus anatomy with hypoplasia or aplasia of the frontal or sphenoid sinuses is found in >50% of adult patients with PCD [21] (Fig. 12.3). Hypertrophy of the inferior turbinate is also a characteristic finding on CT sinuses (Fig. 12.4).

Fig. 12.4 Hypertrophy of inferior turbinates. The inferior turbinates appear as a "sack of potatoes" on the nasal floor

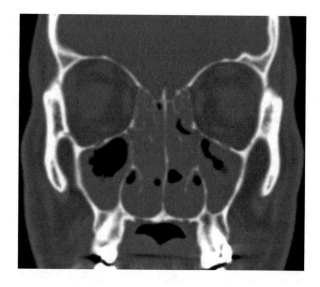

Medical Management

Systemic Medical Therapy

CRS management in general and also in PCD focuses on controlling symptoms and improving quality of life. Systemic therapeutic options include systemic corticosteroids and long-term antibiotics. Systemic corticosteroids may be indicated in the patients with chronic rhinosinusitis with polyposis when the disease is uncontrolled on topical treatment alone. Corticosteroids can control the inflammatory response, reduce polyp size, and alleviate CRS symptoms, but there is a risk of severe side effects, including growth suppression in children and osteoporosis in adulthood. The role of corticosteroids in PCD has not been investigated. Long-term medical therapy with macrolides has proven effective in treating chronic rhinosinusitis without nasal polyposis, especially in patients with normal serum IgE levels [22], and may thus be beneficial in treating PCD patients with CRS as well. This is currently being investigated by an international consortium of PCD investigators (best-cilia.eu).

Topical Medical Therapy

Indisputably, in PCD patients with impaired mucociliary clearance and mucus stagnation, sinonasal irrigation with saline seems to be a safe method for assisting upper airway clearance. Although no studies have evaluated its effect specifically in PCD, it is unlikely to have a detrimental effect.

Airway inflammation in PCD is dominated by neutrophilic infiltration, and therefore, it remains unclear if topical intranasal corticosteroids play a role in the management of PCD CRS. However, given that they are generally well tolerated with few local side effects (such as epistaxis and nasal discomfort) in combination with their excellent safety profile and low systemic absorption, it may be indicated to include nasal steroid spray in a trial of maximal medical therapy before considering surgical intervention. However, inhalation corticosteroid therapy for the treatment of lower airway inflammation is not recommended in PCD, except in patients with overlapping atopic disease [5]. Future studies are required to assess the efficacy of topical intranasal corticosteroids for PCD CRS.

Surgical Management

Only one prospective study has evaluated the outcomes of sinus surgery in PCD [23]. The authors advocated for comprehensive sinus surgery with complete opening of all the paranasal sinuses and removal of all sinus partitions, as pathogens such as *Pseudomonas aeruginosa* can be identified in all sinus cavities (Fig. 12.5). No studies have evaluated the role of mega-antrostomies, medial maxillectomy, or gravity-dependent surgery in PCD.

The authors demonstrated that sinus surgery in combination with extensive rhinologic follow-up and 14 days of systemic antibiotic treatment could eradicate sinus bacteria, reduce pulmonary infections, and improve quality of life for at least 12 months after surgery. More prospective studies from other institutions are needed to confirm these results.

Besides the abovementioned study, only a few retrospective case studies and series have evaluated the effects of sinus surgery in PCD. Generally, they

Fig. 12.5 Endoscopic sinus surgery in a patient with PCD. Mucosal abscesses with growth of *P. aeruginosa* or coagulase-negative staphylococci are common findings

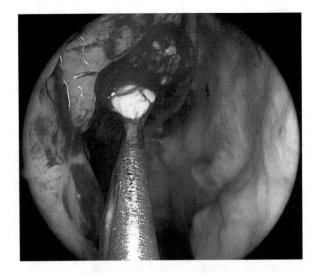

Table 12.1 ESS studies in PCD (including case reports and case series)

Author	Year	No. of PCD patients	Design	Surgical management	Postoperative treatment	Outcome
Mygind and Pedersen [20]	1983	27	Retrospective	Puncture of the sinuses or the Caldwell-Luc procedure	None	Subjective benefit after Caldwell-Luc No effect of sinus punctures
Parsons and Greene [24]	1993	3	Retrospective	Patient 1: antrostomy and anterior ethmoidectomy Patients 2 and 3: antrostomy and total spheno-ethmoidectomy	Intravenous gamma globulin in one patient	Decreased hospitalization and medicine use Subjective benefit
Fakhri et al. [25]	2001	2	Retrospective	ESS. No details	None	Subjective benefit
Berlucchi et al. [22]	2010	1	Case study	Removal of mucocele, antrostomy, and anterior ethmoidectomy	None reported	No pneumonia after surgery
Alanin et al. [26]	2015	8	Retrospective	Comprehensive sinus surgery with opening to all the sinuses		Eradication of sinus bacteria
Alanin et al. [23]	2017	24	Prospective	Comprehensive sinus surgery with opening to all the sinuses	Nasal irrigation, topical steroids, systemic antibiotics	Improved quality of life (SNOT-22) Fewer lung infections
Bequignon et al. [20]	2019	41	Retrospective	Ethmoidectomy eventual turbinate reduction	Not reported	Less facial pain. No improvement in rhinorrhea

consistently demonstrate positive effects, and surgery appears to be a safe and effective treatment options in patients who have failed medical therapy (Table 12.1).

Case Presentation

A 22-year-old female with PCD was referred to ENT due to lung infection with *P. aeruginosa* and severe symptoms of CRS recalcitrant to medical therapy. She reported nasal congestion, thick sticky nasal mucus, facial pressure, and posterior nasal drip that caused nocturnal coughing.

On examination, nasal endoscopy revealed bilateral grade II polyps. The SNOT-22 score was 60. A CT scan of the sinuses demonstrated aplasia of both the frontal and sphenoid sinuses, while there was opacification of the maxillary and ethmoid sinuses. Endoscopic sinus surgery (ESS) with mega-antrostomies to the maxillary sinuses, and a total ethmoidectomy was performed. Bronchoscopy during the same anesthesia was completed. Sinus and lung secretions were cultured, and both grew *P. aeruginosa*.

Postoperative treatment included nasal douching with saline, nasal rinses with colistin, topical nasal steroids, and 2 weeks of intravenous antibiotics. The SNOT-22 score at the 6 and 12 months follow-up was 31 and 22, respectively.

Both pre- and post-ESS monthly sputum samples were routinely cultured. One year prior to ESS, 100% of the cultures grew *P. aeruginosa*. One year following ESS, only 50% of sinus cultures were positive. This case demonstrates that ESS in combination with medical therapy can reduce symptoms of CRS and reduce lung colonization for at least 1 year. In addition, it demonstrates that the sinuses may function as a bacterial reservoir for recurrent lung infections.

Conclusion

PCD is an autosomal recessive inherited genetic disease. CRS is nearly ubiquitous in PCD patients of all ages. Severe nasal polyps in a child should lead the clinician to consider a diagnosis of PCD or CF. Measurement of nasal nitric oxide is a useful screening method; however, definitive diagnosis requires a combination of tests. Medical treatment of PCD CRS may include nasal irrigation with saline, topical nasal steroids, and long-term treatment with macrolide antibiotics. However, randomized controlled studies are lacking. Endoscopic sinus surgery is a safe treatment option for CRS when medical treatment fails. Combined ESS with medical treatment can improve quality of life, eradicate sinus bacteria, and reduce pulmonary colonization in selected patients.

References

1. Siewert AK. Ubereinen fall von bronchiectasis bei einem patienten mit situs inversus viscerum. Berliner Klinische Wochenschrift. 1904;41:139–41.
2. Kartagener M. Zur Pathogenese der Bronchiektasien. Bronchiektasien bei Situs viscerum inversus. Beiträger Klinik der Tuberkulose. 1933;83:489–501.
3. Afzelius BA. A human syndrome caused by immotile cilia. Science. 1976;193(4250):317–9.
4. Sleigh MA. Primary ciliary dyskinesia. Lancet Lond Engl. 1981;2(8244):476.
5. Barbato A, Frischer T, Kuehni CE, Snijders D, Azevedo I, Baktai G, et al. Primary ciliary dyskinesia: a consensus statement on diagnostic and treatment approaches in children. Eur Respir J. 2009;34(6):1264–76.

6. Ferkol TW, Puffenberger EG, Lie H, Helms C, Strauss KA, Bowcock A, et al. Primary ciliary dyskinesia-causing mutations in Amish and Mennonite communities. J Pediatr. 2013;163(2):383–7.

7. Werner C, Onnebrink JG, Omran H. Diagnosis and management of primary ciliary dyskinesia. Cilia. 2015;4(1):2.

8. Davis SD, Ferkol TW, Rosenfeld M, Lee H-S, Dell SD, Sagel SD, et al. Clinical features of childhood primary ciliary dyskinesia by genotype and ultrastructural phenotype. Am J Respir Crit Care Med. 2015;191(3):316–24.

9. Prulière-Escabasse V, Coste A, Chauvin P, Fauroux B, Tamalet A, Garabedian E-N, et al. Otologic features in children with primary ciliary dyskinesia. Arch Otolaryngol Head Neck Surg. 2010;136(11):1121–6.

10. Frija-Masson J, Bassinet L, Honoré I, Dufeu N, Housset B, Coste A, et al. Clinical characteristics, functional respiratory decline and follow-up in adult patients with primary ciliary dyskinesia. Thorax. 2017;72(2):154–60.

11. Noone PG, Leigh MW, Sannuti A, Minnix SL, Carson JL, Hazucha M, et al. Primary ciliary dyskinesia: diagnostic and phenotypic features. Am J Respir Crit Care Med. 2004;169(4):459–67.

12. Shah A, Shoemark A, MacNeill SJ, Bhaludin B, Rogers A, Bilton D, et al. A longitudinal study characterising a large adult primary ciliary dyskinesia population. Eur Respir J [Internet]. 2016 Aug [Cited 2020 Jan 8];48(2):441–50. Available from: http://erj.ersjournals.com/lookup/doi/10.1183/13993003.00209-2016

13. Goutaki M, Meier AB, Halbeisen FS, Lucas JS, Dell SD, Maurer E, et al. Clinical manifestations in primary ciliary dyskinesia: systematic review and meta-analysis. Eur Respir J. 2016;48(4):1081–95.

14. O'Callaghan C, Chilvers M, Hogg C, Bush A, Lucas J. Diagnosing primary ciliary dyskinesia. Thorax. 2007;62(8):656–7.

15. Andersen TN, Alanin MC, von Buchwald C, Nielsen LH. A longitudinal evaluation of hearing and ventilation tube insertion in patients with primary ciliary dyskinesia. Int J Pediatr Otorhinolaryngol. 2016;89:164–8.

16. Sommer JU, Schäfer K, Omran H, Olbrich H, Wallmeier J, Blum A, et al. ENT manifestations in patients with primary ciliary dyskinesia: prevalence and significance of otorhinolaryngologic co-morbidities. Eur Arch Otorhinolaryngol [Internet]. 2011 [Cited 2020 Jan 8];268(3):383–8. Available from: http://link.springer.com/10.1007/s00405-010-1341-9

17. Min YG, Shin JS, Choi SH, Chi JG, Yoon CJ. Primary ciliary dyskinesia: ultrastructural defects and clinical features. Rhinology. 1995;33(4):189–93.

18. Boon M, Smits A, Cuppens H, Jaspers M, Proesmans M, Dupont LJ, et al. Primary ciliary dyskinesia: critical evaluation of clinical symptoms and diagnosis in patients with normal and abnormal ultrastructure. Orphanet J Rare Dis. 2014;9:11.

19. Alanin MC, Nielsen KG, von Buchwald C, Skov M, Aanaes K, Høiby N, et al. A longitudinal study of lung bacterial pathogens in patients with primary ciliary dyskinesia. Clin Microbiol Infect [Internet]. 2015 [Cited 2020 Jan 8];21(12):1093.e1–7. Available from: https://linkinghub.elsevier.com/retrieve/pii/S1198743X1500806X

20. Bequignon E, Dupuy L, Escabasse V, Zerah-Lancner F, Bassinet L, Honoré I, et al. Follow-up and management of chronic rhinosinusitis in adults with primary ciliary dyskinesia: review and experience of our reference centers. J Clin Med. 2019;8(9):1495.

21. Pifferi M, Bush A, Caramella D, Di Cicco M, Zangani M, Chinellato I, et al. Agenesis of paranasal sinuses and nasal nitric oxide in primary ciliary dyskinesia. Eur Respir J. 2011;37(3):566–71.

22. Fokkens WJ, Lund VJ, Mullol J, Bachert C, Alobid I, Baroody F, et al. EPOS 2012: European position paper on rhinosinusitis and nasal polyps 2012. A summary for otorhinolaryngologists. Rhinology. 2012;50(1):1–12.

23. Alanin MC, Aanaes K, Høiby N, Pressler T, Skov M, Nielsen KG, et al. Sinus surgery can improve quality of life, lung infections, and lung function in patients with primary ciliary dyskinesia. Int Forum Allergy Rhinol. 2017;7(3):240–7.

24. Parsons DS, Greene BA. A treatment for primary ciliary dyskinesia: efficacy of functional endoscopic sinus surgery. Laryngoscope. 1993;103(11 Pt 1):1269–72.
25. Fakhri S, Manoukian JJ, Souaid JP. Functional endoscopic sinus surgery in the paediatric population: outcome of a conservative approach to postoperative care. J Otolaryngol. 2001;30(1):15–8.
26. Alanin MC, Johansen HK, Aanaes K, Høiby N, Pressler T, Skov M, et al. Simultaneous sinus and lung infections in patients with primary ciliary dyskinesia. Acta Otolaryngol (Stockh). 2015;135(1):58–63.

Index

© Springer Nature Switzerland AG 2020
D. A. Gudis, R. J. Schlosser (eds.), *The Unified Airway*,
https://doi.org/10.1007/978-3-030-50330-7

Printed in the United States
by Baker & Taylor Publisher Services